Pocket Guide to
Electrocardiography

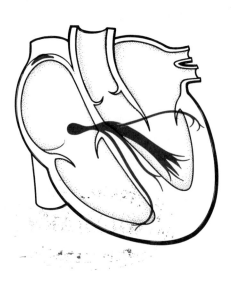

Pocket Guide to
Electrocardiography

Mary Boudreau Conover R.N., B.S.

Director of Education
Critical Care Conferences
Santa Cruz, California

FOURTH EDITION

with **241** illustrations

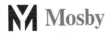

M Mosby

St. Louis Baltimore Boston Carlsbad
Chicago Minneapolis New York Philadelphia Portland
London Milan Sydney Tokyo Toronto

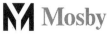

Mosby
Dedicated to Publishing Excellence

A Times Mirror
Company

Publisher: Nancy Coon
Editor: Barry Bowlus
Associate Developmental Editor: Cindi Anderson
Project Manager: John Rogers
Production Editor: Helen Hudlin
Designer: Yael Kats

FOURTH EDITION

Copyright © 1998 by Mosby–Year Book, Inc.

A Mosby imprint of Mosby–Year Book, Inc.

Printed in the United States of America

Mosby–Year Book, Inc.
11830 Westline Industrial Drive
St. Louis, Missouri 64146

Library of Congress Cataloging-in-Publication Data

Conover, Mary Boudreau.
    Pocket guide to electrocardiography / Mary Boudreau Conover.
4th ed.
        p.   cm.
    Includes bibliographical references and index.
    ISBN 0-8151-3695-1 (pbk.)
    1. Electrocardiography–Handbooks, manuals, etc.   2. Arrhythmia–
Diagnosis–Handbooks, manuals, etc.   3. Cardiovascular emergencies–
Diagnosis–Handbooks, manuals, etc.   I. Title.
    [DNLM: 1. Arrhythmia–diagnosis–handbooks.
2. Electrocardiography–handbooks.   3. Electrocardiography–nurses'
instruction.   WG 39 C753p 1998]
RC683.5.E5C646   1998
616.1'207547–dc21
DNLM/DLC
for Library of Congress   97-39597
                                                          CIP

98 99 00 01 02 / 9 8 7 6 5 4 3 2 1

Dedicated to
My brother, **John Boudreau**
and his wife,
Sue Josephson Boudreau

Preface

This pocket book of electrocardiography places the diagnosis and treatment of arrhythmias and cardiac emergencies at your fingertips. As an outlined version of its sister text, *Understanding Electrocardiography,* this pocket edition covers the 12 lead ECG and arrhythmias. It allows you to carry with you a reference for study of ECG recognition, mechanism, pathophysiology, clinical implications, pediatric considerations, bedside diagnosis, emergency treatment, and long term cures.

Because of important new information regarding its mechanism and cure, atrial flutter has been given its own chapter, as has atrial fibrillation, itself under intense and hopeful study in search of a nonsurgical cure.

This compact book provides up-to-date guidelines for emergency and critical care personnel that result in swift ECG diagnosis and correct response for the best possible patient outcome and personal professional pride and confidence.

Mary Boudreau Conover

Abbreviations

APE	acute pulmonary embolism
AV	atrioventricular
AVNR	AV nodal reentry
AVNRT	AV nodal reentry tachycardia
BBB	bundle branch block
CMT	circus movement tachycardia (that associated with WPW syndrome)
LAD	left anterior descending (coronary artery)
LBB	left bundle branch
LBBB	left bundle branch block
LV	left ventricle; left ventricular
MI	myocardial infarction
PAC	premature atrial complex (beat)
PJC	premature junctional complex (beat)
PSVT	paroxysmal supraventricular tachycardia
PVC	premature ventricular complex (beat)
RBB	right bundle branch
RBBB	right bundle branch block
RCA	right coronary artery
RV	right ventricle; right ventricular
SVT	supraventricular tachycardia
Td	torsade(s) de pointes
VA	ventriculoatrial
VT	ventricular tachcyardia
WPW	Wolff-Parkinson-White (syndrome)

Contents

The 12 Electrocardiogram Leads

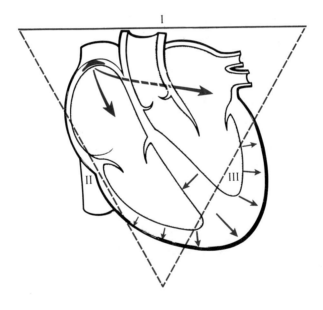

Terminology

Electrocardiograph. A machine that records the electrical activity of the heart.

Electrocardiogram (ECG). The record of the electrical activity of the heart.

ECG lead. Two electrodes of opposite polarity attached to an amplifier within an oscilloscope or strip recorder.

1

Bipolar lead. Two electrodes (+ and −) about equidistant from the heart that contribute equally to the tracing.

Unipolar lead. A positive electrode and an indifferent reference point; the electrical potentials recorded by the positive electrode are compared to the zero reference point. Thus, the contribution is mainly by the positive electrode.

Lead axis. An imaginary line drawn between two electrodes or between a positive electrode and a reference point; all currents generated by the heart relate to this line.

The 12 Leads

There are six limb leads, three bipolar and three unipolar, and six precordial leads (unipolar) in the standard 12-lead ECG. The limb leads provide information about right, left, inferior, or superior current flow. The precordial leads provide information about anterior, posterior, right, and left forces.

Three Bipolar Limb Leads (Einthoven's Triangle)

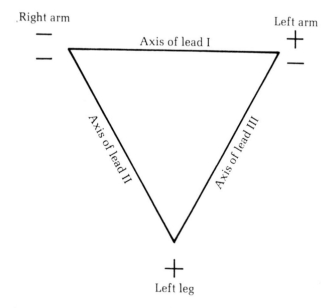

Three bipolar limb leads constitute Einthoven's triangle.
- Lead I: Right arm negative; left arm positive.
- Lead II: Right arm negative; left leg positive.
- Lead III: Left arm negative; left leg positive.

If the two arm electrodes and the left leg electrode of Einthoven's triangle are connected to a central terminal through resistances, the sum of the potentials is virtually zero, the reference point for the unipolar leads.

The Three Unipolar Limb Leads (aVR, aVL, aVF)

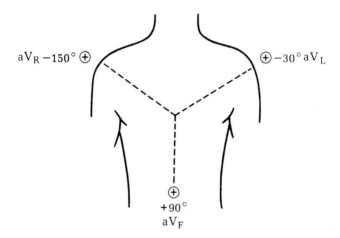

Unipolar limb leads consist of a positive exploring electrode on three limbs (right arm [R], left arm [L], and left leg [F]) paired with the indifferent reference point (center of the heart) from Einthoven's triangle.

Precordial Leads (V_1 to V_6)

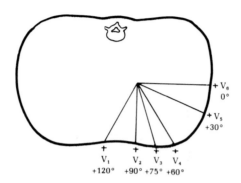

The six principal precordial leads, V_1 to V_6, are unipolar leads, whose axes span from the positive electrodes on the chest wall to the indifferent reference point in Einthoven's triangle. The positive electrode position is as follows:

- V_1 and V_2: Either side of the sternum; fourth intercostal space
- V_4: Midclavicular line; fifth intercostal space
- V_3: Halfway between V_2 and V_4
- V_5 and V_6: The same level with V_4; anterior and midaxillary lines, respectively

Right Chest Leads; Position of Positive Electrode

- V_{3R}: Halfway between V_{4R} and V_1
- V_{4R}: Midclavicular line; fifth intercostal space; right chest
- V_{5R} and V_{6R}: Same level with V_{4R}; anterior and midaxillary lines, respectively

MCL1 and MCL6

The MCL leads are modified (M) versions of the old bipolar chest (C) lead, CL. The modifications consist in placing the negative electrode at the left (L) shoulder, instead of the left arm, and the positive electrode at the V1-6 positions on the precordium. Thus you have the possibilities of MCL1-6.

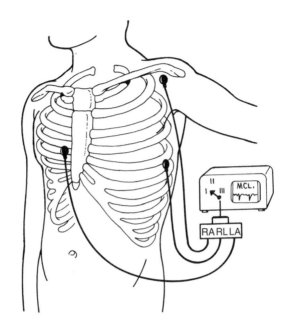

MCL$_1$ and MCL$_6$: Electrodes at V$_1$, V$_6$, and left shoulder

1. Attach the right arm (RA) cable to the left shoulder electrode, left arm (LA) cable to the V$_1$ electrode, and right leg (RL) cable to the V$_6$ electrode.
2. Turn the lead selector to lead I (records MCL$_1$ [simulated V$_1$]).
3. Turn the lead selector to lead II (records MCL$_6$ [simulated V$_6$]).
4. To record a simulated V$_2$ or V$_3$:
   • Move the electrode at the right sternal border to the desired position and turn the lead selector to lead I.
   • Or move the V$_6$ electrode to the desired position and turn the lead selector to lead II.

Placement of Electrodes for Multichannel Monitoring

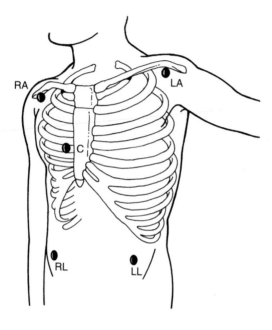

The limb leads and any one precordial lead can be recorded using these electrode positions.

Normal Electrical Activation of the Heart

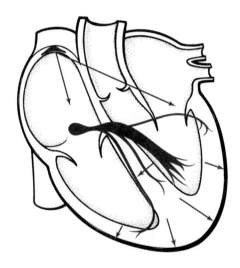

Normal activation of the heart is initiated by the sinus node at a rate consistent with the needs of the body. Atrial activation follows and is from superior to inferior, right to left. The impulse reaches the compact atrioventricular (AV) node first via the fast AV nodal pathway before atrial activation is completed. It is then conducted down the His bundle into the ventricles via the bundle branches and Purkinje fibers. Currents activate both ventricles simultaneously from endocardium to epicardium.

The AV Node and AV Nodal Pathways

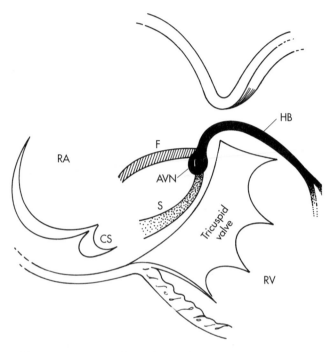

The compact AV node with its fast (anterior) and slow (posterior) fibers. The slow pathway fibers extend from a broad area near the os of the coronary sinus and converge as a common pathway as they reach the compact AV node. The fast pathway fibers arise near the tendon of Todaro and enter the compact AV node superiorly. RA, Right atrium; CS, coronary sinus; AVN, atrioventricular node; F, fast pathway; S, slow pathway; HB, His bundle.
Adapted from Keim S, Werner P, Jazayeri M et al: *Circulation* 86:919, 1992.

The *slow AV nodal fibers* are thought to extend from the coronary sinus os region anteriorly along the tricuspid annulus to join the compact AV node. The *fast AV nodal fibers* are located superiorly along the compact AV node and exit into the atrial septum near Todaro's tendon.

Cellular Electrophysiology

Depolarization: The process by which a resting cell becomes more positive.

Repolarization: The process by which a depolarized cell is restored to its negatively charged resting state.

Resting phase: That time during the cardiac cycle when the myocardial cell is electrically stable at about −90 mV.

Sodium-potassium ATPase pump: An electrogenic transporter; for every enzyme cycle, one molecule of ATP is hydrolyzed, and in a ping-pong fashion, three Na^+ are transported to the outside of the cell in exchange for two K^+.

Action potential: The transmembrane potential of a single cell during the cardiac cycle.

Nonpacemaker cell action potential

The different phases of the action potential shown represent rapid depolarization (phase 0), initial repolarization (phase 1), the plateau (phase 2), rapid repolarization (phase 3), and quiescence (phase 4).

Automaticity: The ability of a cell to depolarize itself, reach threshold potential, and produce a propagated action potential.

Pacemaker cell action potential

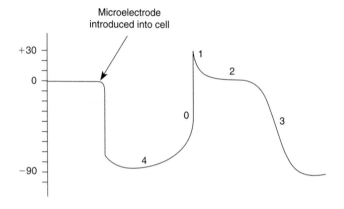

The property of automaticity (phase 4 depolarization) can be seen; note the slow rise of phase 4 as it becomes less and less negative. When threshold potential (−70 mV) is reached, rapid depolarization results.

Step-by-Step Electrical Activation of the Heart (Lead I)

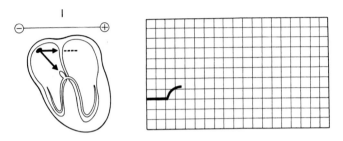

The first half of the *P wave* is inscribed in lead I when the sinus impulse activates the right atrium.

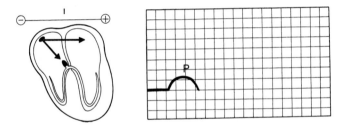

The left atrium and AV node have been activated by the time the P wave is completed. Normally the P wave is smooth in contour.

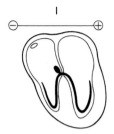 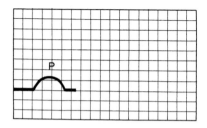

During the *PR segment* (end of the P wave to the beginning of the ventricular complex), the His-Purkinje system is activated (not seen on the surface ECG).

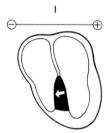 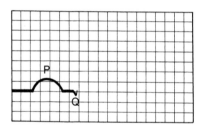

Activation of the IV septum from left to right produces a small, narrow negative deflection *(q wave)* in lead I.

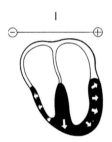 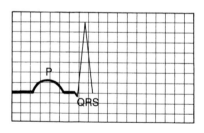

The steep spike of the ventricular complex (QRS) reflects activation of the walls of the heart; the larger left ventricle dominates.

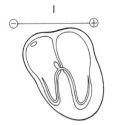 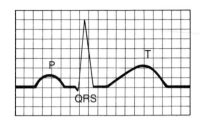

The electrical currents generated during repolarization of the ventricles are reflected in the *ST segment* and the *T wave.* The ST segment is the horizontal line that rises into a slightly asymmetrical curve (the T wave).

The ECG Waveforms and Intervals

3

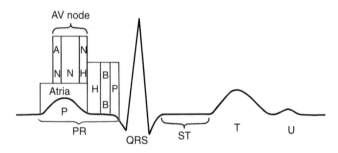

The normal ECG: P wave, atrial depolarization; QRS, ventricular depolarization; ST segment and T wave, ventricular repolarization. The U wave is a small positive deflection. The PR interval reflects not only atrial depolarization, but also the conduction time through the AV node, His bundle (H), bundle branches (BB), and Purkinje fibers (P).

AN, Atrionodal; N, compact AV node; NH, nodal His.

P Wave

- Mechanism: Atrial depolarization
- Duration: Not over 0.11 sec
- Amplitude: Not more than 3 mm
- Polarity:
  1. Positive in I, II, aVF, and V_4 to V_6
  2. Negative in aVR
  3. Positive, negative, or diphasic in III, aVL, and V_1 to V_3; if diphasic, the negative component is last and not excessively broad or deep

- Axis: About +60 degrees in the frontal plane
- Shape: Smooth, not notched or peaked
- Clinical significance of P wave abnormalities
    1. Increased width and notching: left atrial abnormality or right atrial hypertrophy
    2. Increased amplitude: possible atrial enlargement and AV valvular problems, hypertension, cor pulmonale, or congenital heart disease
    3. Diphasic with negative component excessively wide in II or V_1: left atrial enlargement
    4. Peaking that is taller in I than III: right atrial overload
    5. Absent P waves: sinoatrial block, atrial standstill, junctional rhythm with hidden P waves
    6. Inverted P wave where it should be upright: ectopic atrial beats from low in the atria, retrograde activation from junctional beats, or an AV reentry mechanism

QRS Complex

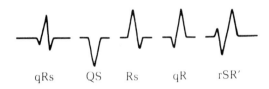

qRs   QS   Rs   qR   rSR′

- Mechanism: Ventricular depolarization
- Duration: Adult, 0.05 to 0.10 sec; newborn, 0.04 to 0.05 sec
- Best leads for measuring: V_1 or V_2
- Amplitude:
    1. Varies with age (greater in the young)
    2. Greater if thin chest walls
    3. Less in obese and in those with lung disease
    4. In precordial leads not less than
        6 mm in V_1 and V_6
        8 mm in V_2 and V_5
        10 mm in V_3 and V_4
    Upper limit of normal is 25 to 30 mm.

5. In bipolar limb leads, too low if the total value (add the positive and negative components) is less than 6 mm in leads I, II, and III.
- Polarity:
  Leads I, II, and V_3 to V_6: positive to equiphasic
  Leads aVL and aVF: positive, negative, or equiphasic
  Lead aVR: negative
- Initial forces (septal)
    Narrow q or 1 to 2 mm in I, aVL, and V_6
    Narrow r in V_1 may normally be absent
- Terminal forces
    S in V_1
    R in V_6
- Axis: −30 to +120 degrees in the frontal plane
- Shape:
  1. The size of each component is indicated by uppercase and lowercase letters. *QRS* is a generic term.
  2. Positive components are R or r waves. If there are two R (or r) waves in the same complex, the second is designated *prime* (R′ or r′).
  3. A negative component is either Q or q (before first R) or S or s (follows an R).
  4. Normal Q wave: less than 0.04 sec and less than 25% the amplitude of the R wave; leads I, aVL, and V_6.
- Clinical significance of QRS abnormalities
  1. Excessive width: intraventricular conduction problems.
  2. Excessive height: ventricular hypertrophy or enlargement.
  3. Low voltage: diffuse coronary disease, cardiac failure, pericardial effusion, myxedema, primary amyloidosis, emphysema, obesity, generalized edema.
  4. The presence or absence of Q waves is judged in the clinical setting.

T Wave

- Mechanism: ventricular repolarization (phase 3 of the action potential)
- Amplitude: not more than 5 mm in limb leads and 10 mm in precordial leads
- Polarity:

1. Positive in I, II, and V_3 to V_6
2. Negative in aVR
3. Positive in aVL and aVF, but may be negative if QRS is less than 6 mm
4. Varies in III, V_1, and V_2

- Shape: Rounded and asymmetrical (notching normal in children), ascending more slowly than it descends
- Vulnerable period

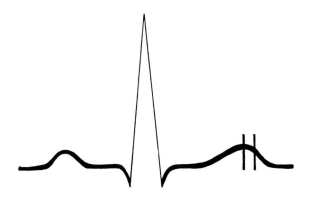

Approximate location of the vulnerable period.

The vulnerable period is at the peak of the T wave, offset slightly toward the end of the T wave. During this short time not all the fibers of the heart are refractory; some are able to accept a stimulus and produce a propagated impulse. The result may be electrical chaos when the current meets with fibers that are still refractory or conducting too slowly.

- Clinical significance of T wave abnormalities
  1. Isolated inversion in asymptomatic adults: usually a normal variant.
  2. Inversion with symptoms: may be diffuse myocardial ischemia or subendocardial infarction.
  3. Following broad QRS: T polarity opposes QRS polarity.
  4. In unstable angina: Progressive deep symmetrical T wave inversion without loss of R waves in precordial lead. Little or no CK or ST elevation is a sign of reperfusion and indicates

critical proximal left anterior descending coronary artery stenosis.

5. Notching: other than in children may indicate pericarditis.
6. Tall and pointed: hyperkalemia, myocardial ischemia, ventricular overload.
7. T wave alternans: hypokalemia, hypocalcemia, hypomagnesemia, tachycardia, congestive heart disease, pericardial disease.
8. Bumps or humps near the apex or on the descending limb of upright T waves: may suggest the long QT syndrome trait in symptomatic blood relatives with borderline QTc interval (corrected for heart rate).

ST Segment

- Mechanism: Early stage of ventricular repolarization
- Polarity:
  1. May be elevated slightly (1 mm) in I, II, and III and as much as 2 mm in some precordial leads
  2. Not depressed more than 0.5 mm in any lead, but may be depressed as much as 4 mm in precordial leads in young black men (early repolarization syndrome)
- J-point: Where the QRS ends and the ST segment begins
- Evaluating displacement: Draw a straight line from J point to J point in sequential cycles
- Shape: Curves very slightly into the beginning of the T wave
- Clinical significance of ST displacement
  1. Significant displacement: coronary artery disease.
  2. Marked elevation: myocardial infarction.
  3. Depression in 8 leads with slight ST elevation in aVR and V_1: left main or three-vessel disease.
  4. Marked depression at rest: myocardial ischemia or subendocardial infarction.
  5. Depression during stress test: Occult coronary artery disease.
  6. Absolutely horizontal ST segment, which forms a sharp angle with the T wave: highly suggestive of myocardial ischemia.
  7. Digitalis: causes typical depression with QT shortening.
  8. Direct current cardioversion: may result in temporary elevation.

9. Chest pain: computer-assisted 12-lead ECG monitoring for ST segment displacement helps to identify transient periods of silent ischemia.
10. Postangioplasty: computer-assisted 12-lead ECG monitoring for ST displacement alerts to abrupt closure from spasm or thrombus.

- ST elevation and location of the culprit lesion:

  $aVL + V_{2-5}$ = proximal LAD (left anterior descending) before first diagonal coronary artery

  $aVL + V_2$ + isoelectric or depressed ST in V_{3-5} = first diagonal

  aVL + isoelectric or depressed ST in precordial leads = first obtuse marginal

PR Interval

- Mechanism: AV conduction time
- Duration: 0.12 to 0.20 sec
- Measure: From the beginning of the P wave to the first ventricular deflection (Q or R)
- Clinical significance of PR abnormalities
  1. Shortened: sinus tachycardia, preexcitation syndromes, AV junctional rhythms, glycogen storage disease, or hypertension.
  2. Prolonged: sinus bradycardia, AV block, beta blockers, or hypothyroidism.
  3. Note: A PR interval that is shorter or longer than the prescribed limit may be normal for a particular individual.

QT Interval

- Mechanism: Ventricular repolarization time
- Duration: "Rule of thumb" is less than half the preceding RR interval.
- Measure: From the beginning of the ventricular complex to the end of the T wave in a lead where the end of the T wave is best seen (e.g., lead II). After myocardial infarction, the longest QT interval is usually seen in leads V_2 to V_4.
- Normal variations: Significantly influenced by heart rate and autonomic tone; varies in males and females and with age
- Correction for heart rate (QT_c): Usually 0.39 sec plus or minus 0.04 sec at any heart rate. Basett's formula is used and is based on

the observation that the QT interval varies with the square root of the cycle length (divide the square root of the RR interval into the QT interval, measured in seconds). A normal range for the QTc remains unsettled, because a wide range has been observed in normal subjects as well as in individuals with long QT syndrome.

- Clinical significance of QT abnormalities
  1. QT lengthening: idiopathic or drug related (quinidine, procainamide hydrochloride, disopyramide, amiodarone), hypokalemia, hypomagnesemia, cerebrovascular disease, hypothermia, bradycardia.
  2. Prolonged QT reflects dispersion of repolarization within the myocardium, predisposing to a malignant polymorphous ventricular tachycardia known as torsades de pointes. It may be prolonged by 10% to 15% in trained athletes.
  3. Use of QTc: Evaluation of drug effects on ventricular repolarization; construction of rate-adaptive pacemakers; may play a role in prediction of risk after acute myocardial infarction.

U Wave

- Mechanism: Unknown
- Amplitude: Low voltage
- Polarity: Same as the T wave
- Clinical significance of U wave abnormalities
  1. Hypokalemia (tall U wave fusing with T).
  2. Reversed polarity in myocardial ischemia, hypertensive left ventricular overload, aortic or mitral regurgitation, left coronary artery disease (at rest).
  3. Taller in hypokalemia.
  4. Inverted in heart disease.
  5. Hypertension is the most common cause of the initial part of the U wave being negative.
  6. Transient terminal U wave inversion: acute myocardial ischemia.

QRS Complex in the Limb Leads

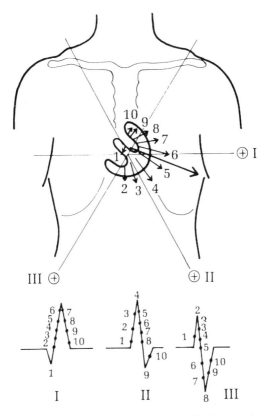

Instant-to-instant cardiac vectors related to the bipolar limb leads. The numbers on the ventricular complexes correspond to the cardiac vectors. Septal activation is well defined in lead I (vector 1).

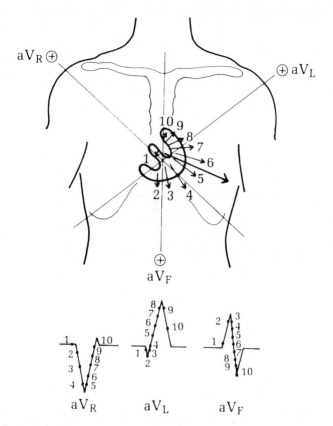

Instant-to-instant cardiac vectors related to the unipolar limb leads. The numbers on the ventricular complexes correspond to the cardiac vectors.

The long arrow represents the electrical axis of the heart; numbers indicate the sequence in which the current arrives at the epicardium. Graph moves up when current is flowing toward a positive electrode and is most positive when the current is parallel with the lead axis. Graph is isoelectric when current is perpendicular to the lead axis. Graph moves down when current is toward the negative electrode.

Normal QRS Complexes in the Precordial Leads

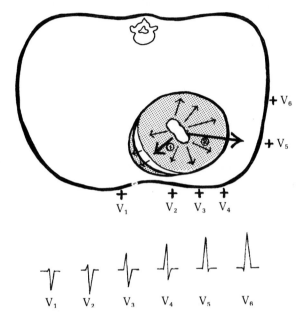

Ventricular activation as seen in the precordial leads. Note the normal R-wave progression.

From V_1 to V_6 the positive electrode gets closer and closer to current flow in the thick-walled left ventricle, and the R wave (positive component) becomes taller and taller. This normal R wave progression reflects intact anterior forces; if anterior forces are lost, so are the R waves. In V_1 the initial little r wave reflects both septal and right ventricular forces. However, when right ventricular activation is still just beginning, the dominant leftward force of the left ventricle produces a deep S wave. Thus, a narrow rS complex is normal for V_1, although the little r wave may be normally absent.

Transitional Zone

Transitional Zones

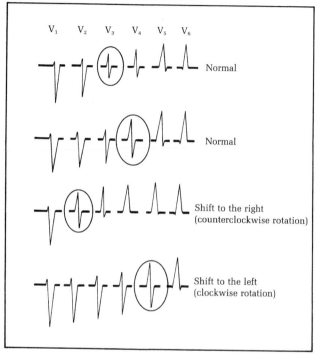

Normal transitional zones (V_3 to V_4) compared with clockwise and counterclockwise rotation of the heart.

Normal: The equiphasic complex is between V_3 and V_4.
Shift to the left (toward V_6): Clockwise rotation of the heart.
Shift to the right (toward V_1): Counterclockwise rotation.

ECG Grid

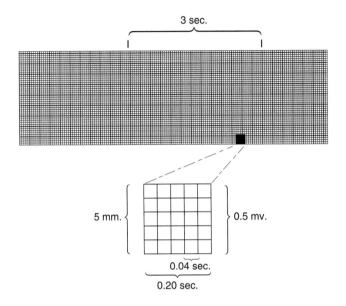

Time is measured on the horizontal plane.

Each small square is 1 mm long and represents 0.04 sec.

Each larger square is 5 mm long and represents 0.2 sec in time when the paper speed is 25 mm/sec.

Amplitude (voltage) is measured on the vertical plane. All diagnostic 12-lead ECGs are standardized so that 1 mV is equal to 10 mm (two large squares). The single vertical lines above the ECG grid are 3 inches apart and represent 3-sec intervals when the paper speed is 25 mm/sec.

Calculation of Heart Rate

If the rhythm is irregular:

Count the number of cycles in a 6-sec strip and multiply by 10.

If the rhythm is regular:

1. Count the number of large squares between two R waves and divide into 300.
2. Measure the time interval in seconds between two R waves and divide into 60.
3. Count the number of small squares (0.04 sec) between R waves (for ventricular rate) or P waves (for atrial rate) and divide into 1,500.

Determination of the Electrical Axis

4

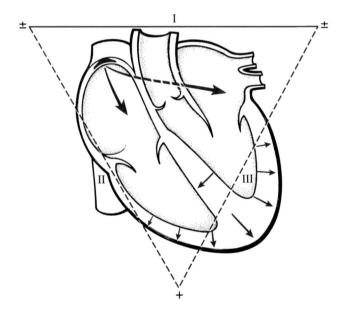

The ability to determine the electrical axis of the heart gives depth to your understanding of the 12-lead ECG and is a necessary skill in the intelligent response to some cardiac emergencies (broad QRS tachycardia, high-risk myocardial infarction, life-threatening hyperkalemia).

Instant-to-Instant Electrical Activation of the Heart

The intraventricular septum is the first to be activated; the impulse then travels from the endocardium to the epicardium, arriving at the thinner-walled right ventricular epicardium first. The ventricular arrows in the heart on p. 27 represent the instant-to-instant cardiac vectors. The activation process in the normal heart takes about 0.08 sec or less. The currents begin in both ventricles at almost the same time. However, activation of the thicker left ventricular wall takes longer.

Axis at a Glance (using leads I and II)

Normal	Left	Extreme left	Right
−30 to +110°	>0°	>−30°	>+120°

The Easy Two-Step (looking for the equiphasic deflection)

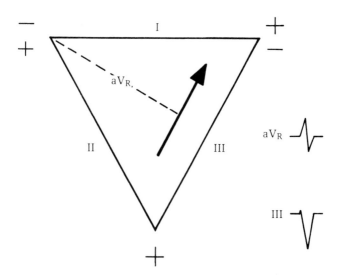

Deflections in leads aV_R and III when the axis is –60 degrees.

Step 1: Look for an equiphasic deflection in the 6 limb leads. In the example it is found in aVR, indicating that the main current flow is perpendicular to the axis of that lead. However, this is incomplete information because the current may be superior or inferior.

Step 2: Look at the lead whose axis is parallel to the current flow; in this case, lead III. Because the complex in III is negative, current is flowing toward the negative electrode of lead III (superiorly). There is left axis deviation of –60 degrees.

Exercise 1: Normal Axis

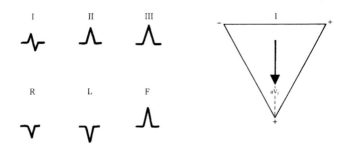

Step 1: The equiphasic deflection is in lead I; therefore, current flow is perpendicular to that lead axis.

Step 2: Look at the complex in the lead whose axis is parallel with the current flow (lead aVF).

Conclusion: Since the complex in lead aVF is positive, current is flowing toward the positive electrode of that lead (inferiorly at +90 degrees).

Exercise 2: No-Man's-Land Axis (northwest quadrant)

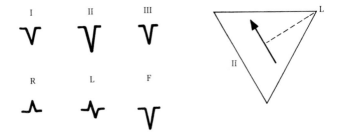

Step 1: The equiphasic deflection is in lead aVL; therefore, current flow is perpendicular to that lead axis.

Step 2: Look at the complex in the lead whose axis is parallel with the current flow (lead II).

Conclusion: Since the complex in lead II is negative, current is flowing toward the negative electrode of that lead (superiorly at −120 degrees).

Exercise 3: Left Axis Deviation

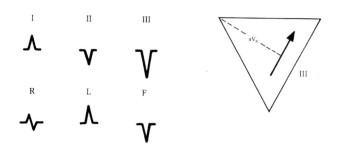

Step 1: The equiphasic deflection is in lead aVR; therefore, current flow is perpendicular to that lead axis.

Step 2: Look at the complex in the lead whose axis is parallel with the current flow (lead III).

Conclusion: Since the complex in lead III is negative, current is flowing toward the negative electrode of that lead (superiorly at −60 degrees).

Exercise 4: Right Axis Deviation

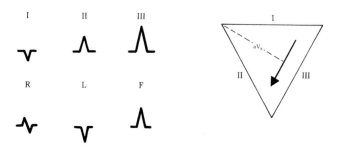

Step 1: The equiphasic deflection is again in lead aVR; therefore, current flow is perpendicular to that lead axis.

Step 2: Look at the complex in the lead whose axis is parallel with the current flow (again, lead III).

Conclusion: Since the complex in lead III is positive this time, current is flowing toward the positive electrode of that lead (inferiorly at +120 degrees).

Quadrant Method (using leads I and aVF)

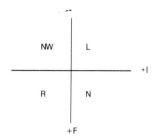

The quadrant method uses the axes of leads I and aVF to divide the thorax into quarters: left (L), normal (N), right (R), and northwest (NW; no man's land).

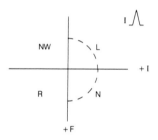

If the complex in lead I is upright, the axis is somewhere in the positive half of lead I.

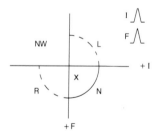

If the complex in lead aVF is also upright, the axis is in the normal quadrant.

Note: Lead aVF can also be used to tell at a glance if the QRS axis is inferior or superior. It is immediately apparent by looking at the figure that a positive QRS complex in aVF is an inferior axis, and a negative complex, a superior axis.

The Hexaxial Figure

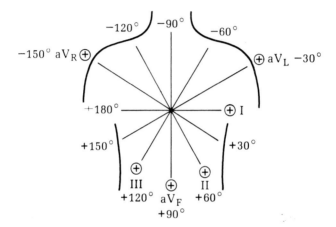

When a more precise determination of axis is needed, the hexaxial figure is used. All frontal plane lead axes are drawn through a central point. Each lead axis is a 30-degree increment with lead I at 0 degrees to the left and plus or minus 180 degrees to the right.

The Mechanisms of Arrhythmias

5

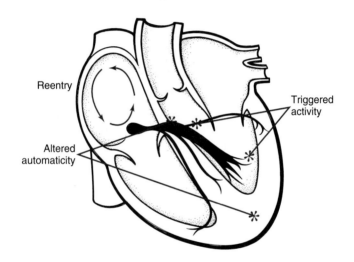

Two Categories of Arrhythmias

1. Abnormalities of conduction (block or reentry)
2. Abnormalities of impulse initiation (abnormal automaticity, enhanced normal automaticity, or triggered activity)

Reentry

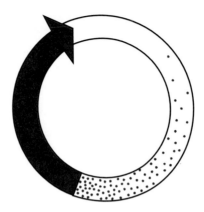

Reentry is the reactivation of fibers for a second time or repeatedly by the same wave front. Slow conduction is usually part of the reentrant pathway. Four types of reentry have been described: anatomic, functional, anisotropic, and reflection.

Anatomic reentry: An excitation wave that passes around an anatomic obstacle or obstacles.

Functional reentry: An excitation wave that does not require an anatomic structure to circle around; it depends on the local differences in conduction velocity.

Anisotropic reentry: A circuit that is determined by the difference in conduction velocities through the length of the fiber versus across its width.

Reflection: Occurs in parallel pathways of Purkinje fibers or myocardial tissues that have depressed segments. The impulse is blocked in the severely depressed segment and transmitted slowly in a less-depressed neighboring fiber to activate surrounding tissue and return retrogradely through the previously blocked segment.

Altered Automaticity

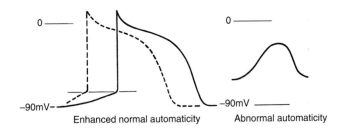

Enhanced normal automaticity   Abnormal automaticity

The two types of altered automaticity are as follows:

Enhanced normal automaticity: A steepening of phase 4 (dashed line) in normal His-Purkinje fibers influenced by catecholamines and resulting in an increased firing rate—about 100 beats/min (rarely faster).

Abnormal automaticity: The spontaneous firing of cardiac cells because of conditions that cause a reduction in membrane potential (e.g., ischemia, infarction, hypokalemia, hypocalcemia, and cardiomyopathy). Areas of abnormal automaticity may easily surface when the rate of the sinus node drops below that of the ectopic focus.

Triggered Activity

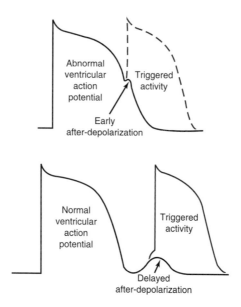

Triggered activity is an arhythmogenic mechanism caused by early or delayed afterdepolarizations that produce premature beats and tachycardias.

Afterdepolarizations

Afterdepolarizations are oscillations of membrane potential that attend or follow the action potential and depend on preceding transmembrane activity for their manifestation. When these oscillations depolarize the cell to threshold potential, they induce spontaneous action potentials (triggered activity).

Early afterdepolarization:

Oscillation of the membrane potential during phase 2 and/or phase 3 of the cardiac action potential associated with the class IA drugs (quinidine, procainamide, disopyramide) and with slow heart rates and hypokalemia. (See Chapter 14.)

Delayed afterdepolarization:

Oscillation of the membrane potential following full repolarization associated with drugs such as digitalis that cause increased intracellular levels of calcium. (See Chapter 17.)

Clinical Application

ECG differentiation among the mechanisms of reentry, altered automaticity, and triggered activity is at best difficult and often impossible. However, occasionally ECG clues point to one mechanism or another.

Automaticity is suspected when there is

- Gradual acceleration of an arrhythmia
- Gradual emergence of an arrhythmia
- Long coupling intervals
- Variable coupling intervals
- A fusion beat at the onset of an arrhythmia

Examples of automatic rhythms include parasystole, escape rhythms, nonparoxysmal junctional tachycardia, and accelerated idioventricular rhythms.

Reentry is suspected when there is

- Fixed coupling
- Abrupt onset of tachycardia
- Abrupt termination of tachycardia

Triggered activity is suspected in

- Long-QT VT (torsades de pointes; early afterdepolarizations)
- Tachycardias of digitalis toxicity (delayed afterdepolarizations)

Arrhythmias Originating in the Sinus Node

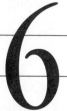

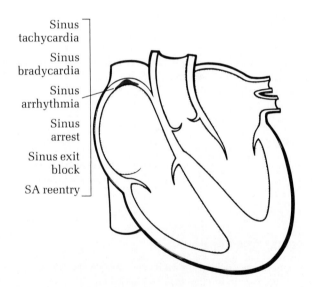

Sinus tachycardia

Sinus bradycardia

Sinus arrhythmia

Sinus arrest

Sinus exit block

SA reentry

The arrhythmias originating in the sinus (sinoatrial [SA] node) are physiological or pathological. The physiological ones are the responses to fever and sympathetic stimulation; the pathological ones are associated with sinus nodal disease.

Anatomy

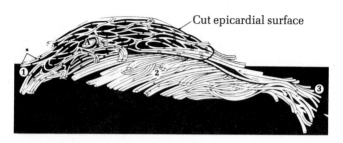

Cut epicardial surface

A wax model of the human sinus node.
From Truex RC. In Wellens HJJ, Lie KI, Hanse MJ, editors: *The conduction system of the heart,* Hingham, Mass, 1976, Martinus Nijhoff.

The sinus node (or sinoatrial node) is located in the wall of the right atrium, adjacent to the superior vena cava. The body of the SA node blends with perinodal fibers, which in turn blend with atrial tissue (1, 2, and 3 in the illustration).

Physiology

The SA node has calcium channel action potentials; thus, conduction velocity through the node is normally slow. The autonomic nervous system controls the discharge rate of the sinus node (decreases with vagal stimulation; increases with sympathetic stimulation).

Normal Sinus Rhythm

A normal sinus rhythm is paced by the SA node at a rate of not less than 60 beats/min or more than 100 beats/min.

ECG Recognition

Rate: 60 to 100 beats/min; be alert to possible problems at heart rates faster than 90 beats/min.
Rhythm: Regular or slightly irregular (effect of respirations).
P wave polarity: Positive in I, II, aVF, and V_4 to V_6; negative in aVR; positive, negative, or biphasic in III, aVL, and V_1 to V_3.
Distinguishing features:
- P waves all the same shape in a single lead.
- Heart rate consistent with the needs of the body.
- Asymptomatic.

Pediatrics

The younger the age, the faster the normal sinus rate.
First week of life: less than 140 beats/min
First year: less than 120 beats/min

Sinus Tachycardia

Sinus tachycardia is the rapid beating of the SA node at a rate of more than 100 beats/min.

ECG Recognition

II

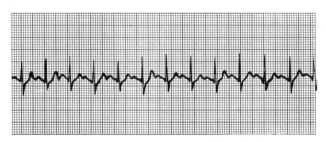

Rate: 100 to 180 beats/min; higher with exertion.
Rhythm: May be slightly irregular; gradual onset and gradual termination.
P waves: Usually identical in shape to the P waves of normal sinus rhythm, although the pacing site within the sinus node may shift, causing the shape of the P wave to differ from that of a slower sinus rhythm.
PR interval: Normal, unless associated with AV block or preexcitation; shortens with increase in heart rate.
QRS complex: Not affected.
QT interval: Shortens.

Mechanism

Physiologically enhanced automaticity (steepening of phase 4 of the action potential) is due to sympathetic stimulation or vagal block.

Causes

- Congestive heart failure
- Cardiogenic shock
- Acute pulmonary embolism
- Acute myocardial infarction
- Infarct extension
- Any condition that increases sympathetic stimulation (exercise, emotion, pain, fever, inflammation)
- Atropine
- Catecholamines
- Thyroid
- Alcohol
- Nicotine
- Caffeine
- Sympathomimetic agents in nose drops

▶ **Clinical Implications**

- May precipitate ventricular arrhythmias in the setting of mitral stenosis or severe ischemia
- Primary sinus node abnormality

Pediatrics

The younger the age of the patient, the faster the heart rate in sinus tachycardia.
Infant: >200 beats/min
Child: between 140 and 200 beats/min

Bedside Diagnosis

- Regular pulse
- Normal neck vein pulsation
- Constant systolic blood pressure
- Constant intensity of first heart sound
- Response to carotid sinus massage:
    Gradual and temporary slowing of heart rate
    PR interval lengthens
    Nonconducted P waves possible
    Accentuated antagonism (the greater the level of sympathetic activity, the more pronounced the effect)

Differential Diagnosis

In atrial tachycardia caused by digitalis toxicity (rate: 130–250 beats/min), the P waves are identical in shape to those of sinus tachycardia. Clues are as follows:
- Clinical setting
- Appropriateness of the tachycardia
- Heart rate
- Presence of AV block (usually 2:1)
- Physical signs of digitalis toxicity

Treatment

There is no treatment, although a physical assessment is indicated. If the rhythm is inappropriate or the patient is symptomatic, the cause should be identified and treated (e.g., for hypovolemia, fever) or eliminated (e.g., for tobacco, alcohol, caffeine).

Sinus Bradycardia

Sinus bradycardia is the slow beating of the sinus node.

ECG Recognition

II

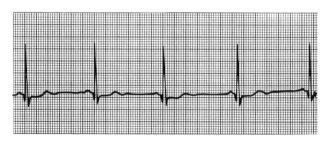

Rate: Less than 60 beats/min in the adult (50 beats/min in an athlete is not abnormal).
Rhythm: Regular unless associated with sinus arrhythmia.
P waves: Identical in shape to the P waves of normal sinus rhythm.
PR interval: Normal, unless associated with AV block or preexcitation. Lengthens with decrease in heart rate.
QRS complex: Not affected.

QT interval: Lengthens

Distinguishing features: Rate, rhythm, and uniform shape of the P
   waves. The slow rate is quickly diagnosed because there are more
   than 5 large squares between R waves.

Mechanisms

- Enhanced vagal tone (normal during sleep)
- Decreased sympathetic tone
- Anatomical changes

Causes

- Sleep
- Athletic heart
- Increased vagal tone or decreased sympathetic tone
- Meningitis
- Increased intracranial pressure
- Cervical or mediastinal tumor
- Hypoxia
- Myxedema
- Hypothermia
- Fibrodegenerative changes
- Gram-negative sepsis
- Mental depression
- Eye surgery
- Coronary arteriography
- Vomiting and vasovagal syncope

▶ Clinical Implications

- Benign in trained athletes.
- Absence during sleep suggests nodal disease.
- Associated syncope indicates severe case.
- Common and possibly beneficial in acute myocardial infarction,
  especially of the inferior wall.
- When profound and associated with hypotension and acute MI, the
  prognosis is poor, especially if the deteriorating hemodynamic
  situation is not corrected rapidly.
- May occur during reperfusion with thrombolytic agents.
- Associated with a poor prognosis if it occurs after resuscitation
  from cardiac arrest.

Pediatrics

Sinus bradycardia is rare in normal healthy children. Neonates can tolerate ventricular rates of 55 beats/min or less with normal hearts and 65 beats/min with congenital heart disease. It is seen in hypothyroidism, hypothermia, hypopituitarism, obstructive jaundice, typhoid fever, normal premature infants, and as a reflex bradycardia in increased intracranial pressure, increased systemic blood pressure, and cardiac catheterization.

Bedside Diagnosis

- Regular pulse.
- Normal neck vein pulsation.
- Constant systolic blood pressure.
- Constant intensity of first heart sound.
- Response to carotid sinus massage: Rate gradually and temporarily slows.
- Response to vagal block: The normal sinus node increases its rate, usually by more than 50% above baseline but not more than 120 beats/min. In fact, one of the signs of intrinsic sinus nodal dysfunction is that the heart rate does not exceed 90 beats/min following vagal block with 2 to 4 mg/kg of atropine IV.

Treatment

None, unless symptomatic, and then atropine (0.5 mg IV initially, and repeated if necessary). A pacemaker may be needed in congestive heart failure or if bradycardia is chronic and associated with low cardiac output.

Sinus Arrhythmia

Sinus arrhythmia is the variation in heart rate that is often synchronized with breathing, slowing with expiration and accelerating with inspiration.

ECG Recognition

II

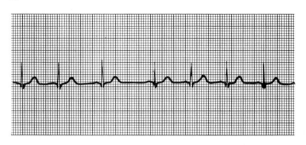

Rate: Slows with expiration; accelerates with inspiration.
Rhythm: Irregular.
P waves: Normal.
PR interval: Not affected.
QRS complex: Not affected.
QT interval: Becomes longer during the slow phase of this rhythm.
Distinguishing features: Rate varies with respiration; cyclical, irregular rhythm; uniform shape of P waves.

Mechanism

The effect of respirations on sinus rhythm is a balance between sympathetic and parasympathetic tone. Normally during sleep, parasympathetic activity predominates. However, in patients with anterior myocardial infarcts, this may be suppressed by the relatively high sympathetic activity, which in turn causes increased susceptibility to ventricular arrhythmias and sudden death.

Causes

In the healthy heart:
• Exercise
• Mental stress
• Respiration
• Blood pressure regulation
• Thermoregulation
• Actions of the renin-angiotensin system
• Circadian rhythms

Other causes:
- Aging
- Postprandial hypotension
- Diabetes
- Alcoholic cardiomyopathy

Symptoms

Uncommon; excessively long pauses may result in dizziness or syncope if not accompanied by an escape rhythm.

Pediatrics

Rare in the young infant; normal in children and adolescents.

Treatment

None, unless symptomatic.

SA Wenckebach (Type I SA Block)

SA Wenckebach is the progressive lengthening of SA conduction until P wave conduction to the atria fails for one beat and sequence begins again.

ECG Recognition

V_1

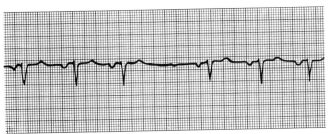

Rate: There may be bradycardia because of the pauses.
Rhythm: Group beating (usually pairs or groups of 3).
P waves: Sinus.
PP intervals: Groups of shortening PPs and a pause.
The pause: Less than twice the shortest cycle.
PR interval: Not affected.

QRS complex: Not affected.

Distinguishing features: Group beating; normal P waves; shortening PP intervals (except with a 3:2 SA conduction ratio); pauses that are less than twice the shortest cycle.

Mechanism

Sinus and AV nodal cells have slow-response action potentials, slow conduction, and similar conduction problems. Although the sinus node is capable of beating very rapidly, the conduction of an impulse through and out of this tissue is always at least as slow as conduction through the AV node.

Causes

- Drugs (e.g., quinidine, procainamide, digitalis)
- Acute myocarditis
- Myocardial infarction
- Fibrosis of the atrium
- Excessive vagal stimulation

▶ Clinical Implications

- Usually transient (ambulatory patients, trained athletes, and healthy young persons)
- May be part of the sick sinus syndrome when associated with other arrhythmias

Pediatrics

SA Wenckebach is seen in infants (especially newborns) and children without heart disease. In adolescents it is usually caused by increased vagal tone.

Treatment

None unless the pauses are symptomatic, and then it is managed as a sinus bradycardia.

Type II SA Block

Type II SA block is the regular firing of the sinus node with periodic failure of SA conduction and fixed PP intervals before and after the pause.

ECG Recognition

II

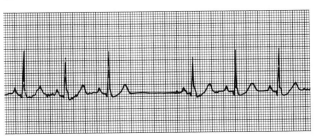

Rate: Pauses in the sinus rhythm may cause bradycardia.
Rhythm: Regular before and after the pauses.
P waves: Sinus.
PP intervals: Fixed before and after the pauses.
PR interval: Normal and fixed unless there is an associated AV conduction problem.
The pause: Can be multiplied by an integer (a whole number).
QRS complex: Not affected.
Distinguishing features: Dropped P waves; fixed PR intervals; pauses that are multiples of the PP intervals.

Sinus Arrest or Sinus Pause

Sinus arrest or sinus pause is a failure of impulse formation in the sinus node.

ECG Recognition

V₁

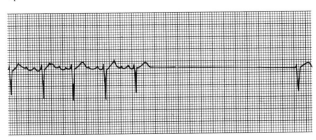

Rate: May be marked bradycardia because of long pauses.

Rhythm: Regular with pauses that have no numerical relationship to the basic cycle length.

P waves: There may be normal sinus P waves along with atrial escape beats.

PP interval: May be fixed before and after the pauses.

The pause: Not a multiple of a whole number.

PR interval: Not affected.

QRS complex: Not affected.

Distinguishing features: A pause in sinus rhythm that is not a multiple of a whole number.

Treatment

None, unless the pauses are symptomatic and complicated by other arrhythmias (sick sinus syndrome). Then a pacemaker may be indicated.

Permanent Atrial Standstill

Permanent atrial standstill is the inability of the atria to respond to stimuli.

ECG Recognition

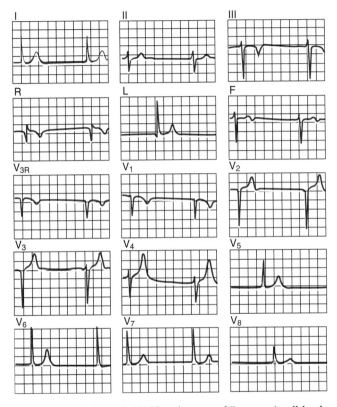

Permanent atrial standstill. The absence of P waves in all leads is evident, including a right precordial lead (V_{3R}) and extreme left precordial leads V_7 and V_8.

(Courtesy Dr. James Wolliscroft, Ann Arbor, Mich.)

P waves: Absent in all leads.

QRS complex: Junctional or ventricular escape beats.

Distinguishing features: Absent P waves (ECG and atrial electrogram).

Mechanism

The atrium is immobile on fluoroscopy and cannot be stimulated electrically. It is possible that the sinus node may actually be firing but that the atrium is incapable of responding.

▶ Clinical Implications

- Long-standing progressive cardiac disease
- Neuromuscular disease

Physical Signs

- Vertigo or syncope
- Absent A waves in jugular venous pulse and right atrium

Treatment

Pacemaker

Sinus Nodal Dysfunction (Sick Sinus Syndrome)

Sick sinus syndrome (SSS) includes disorders of impulse generation and conduction, failure of latent pacemakers, and a susceptibility to paroxysmal or chronic atrial tachycardias.

ECG Recognition

Rate: Too fast, too slow, or both.
Rhythm: Irregular.
P waves: Sinus or atrial.
PR interval: Not affected.
QRS complex: Not affected.
QT interval: Varies with heart rate.
Distinguishing features: Any of the following may be present and associated with syncope:
- Persistent sinus bradycardia
- Sinus pauses or sinus arrest
- SA block
- Episodic atrial fibrillation (with a non–drug-induced slow ventricular response), atrial flutter, and atrial tachycardia
- Bradycardia alternating with tachycardia (usually paroxysmal atrial fibrillation or flutter)
- Inappropriate sinus node response to exercise or stress
- Frequently intermittent and unpredictable

Variations

II

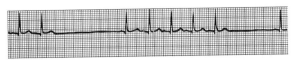

- SSS with Type II second-degree SA block

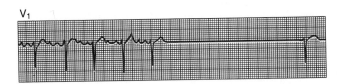

- SSS caused by bradycardia-tachycardia.

(From Marriott HJL, Conover M: *Advanced concepts in arrhythmias,* St Louis, 1983, Mosby.)

II

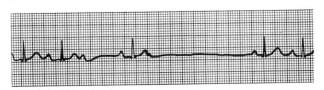

- SSS with inappropriate overdrive suppression after an early premature atrial complex (PAC) (in the T wave before the pause)

Mechanisms

A wide spectrum of abnormalities of both sinus node automaticity and SA conduction cause the long sinus pauses of SSS. Complete SA block with an atrial escape rhythm can occur. After atrial tachyarrhythmias, the long pauses are the result of SA block and overdrive suppression of the sinus node.

Causes

- Cardiac glycosides
- Sympatholytic antihypertensive agents
- β-blockers
- Calcium channel blockers
- Membrane-active antiarrhythmic agents
- Marked hypervagotonia, sometimes combined with certain drugs
- Coronary atherosclerosis
- Partial or total destruction of the SA node
- Discontinuity between the SA node and atrial tissue
- Inflammatory or degenerative processes altering nerve supply

Pediatrics

Seen in children during the postoperative period, usually following extensive intraatrial surgery (especially surgery for transposition of the great vessels). The rhythms seen are as follows:
- Profound sinus bradycardia
- Sinus arrest
- Atrial or junctional rhythms
- Atrial flutter
- Atrial fibrillation (rare)

Treatment

Treatment varies relative to patient's symptoms and ECG:
- Anticoagulation
- Preservation of organized atrial activation
- Chronotropic support for exertional intolerance
- Permanent pacing when syncope is related to bradyarrhythmia

SA Nodal Reentry Tachycardia

SA nodal reentry tachycardia is an uncommon cause of paroxysmal supraventricular tachycardia (PSVT).

ECG Recognition

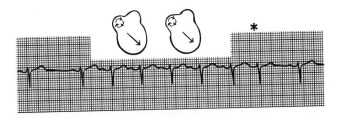

Paroxysmal supraventricular tachycardia (PSVT) resulting from SA nodal reentry. The tachycardia is terminated by a single PAC (in the T wave with the asterisk).

Rate: 80–140 beats/min, often with wide fluctuations.

Rhythm: PSVT (sustained form lasts more than 30 sec).

P waves: Look like sinus P waves.

PR interval: Usually normal and fixed, unless AV block.

QRS complex: Normal unless associated with an intraventricular conduction problem.

Distinguishing features: Often goes unnoticed; may resemble sinus arrhythmia but not influenced by respirations; sinus P waves; terminates with vagal maneuvers or adenosine.

Mechanism

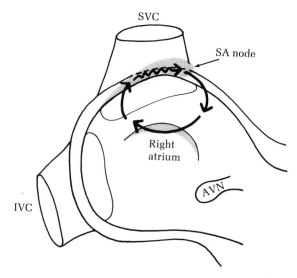

Mechanism of SA nodal reentry tachycardia.

Reentry circuit may be initiated by a PAC or a sinus beat and be completely confined to the sinus node, or it may involve surrounding atrial tissue.

Symptoms

- May go unnoticed or be slightly bothersome
- Palpitations (>50%)
- Angina, dyspnea, and syncope (especially if heart disease or sick sinus syndrome)

Clinical Implications

- May be misdiagnosed as an anxiety-related sinus tachycardia
- Causes may be ischemia or cardiomyopathy

Treatment

- Acute setting: Vagal maneuvers and adenosine
- Long term (cure): Sinus node modification with radiofrequency catheter ablation

Wandering Pacemaker

A wandering pacemaker is a sinus arrhythmia with an escape atrial or junctional rhythm, often resulting in atrial fusion beats.

ECG Recognition

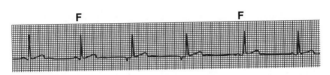

Sinus slowing with a junctional escape rhythm (often called a wandering pacemaker). There is an atrial fusion beat (F) as the two foci (sinus and junctional) vie for control of the heart.

Rate: Bradycardia.
Rhythm: Irregular.
P waves: Multiform with fusion beats.
PR or P′R intervals: Normal unless associated with an AV conduction problem or preexcitation. A P′ wave is an ectopic P wave.
QRS complex: Not affected.
Distinguishing features: Sinus bradycardia with changing P wave shapes.

Mechanism

Sinus slowing occurs, permitting an atrial ectopic focus to escape at a rate of 50 beats/min. During the transition from sinus rhythm to the escape rhythm and back again, both the sinus node and the junction activate the atria at the same time, producing atrial fusion (F) beats.

Clinical Implications

Occurs frequently in normal individuals and is of no consequence.

Treatment

None.

Heart Rate Variability

Heart rate variability is the beat-to-beat variation in heart rate, a marker of autonomic input into the heart. Its measurement requires

Holter monitoring and appropriate computer software. *Baroreflex sensitivity* is another method used to assess autonomic nervous system tone and may be more predictive of cardiac events.

► Clinical Implications

Decreased heart rate variability after acute myocardial infarction indicates abnormalities of baseline parasympathetic tone and is a strong predictor of arrhythmic events and sudden death.

∿ Hypersensitive Carotid Sinus Syndrome

Cardioinhibitory carotid sinus hypersensitivity is ventricular asystole of more than 3 seconds during carotid sinus stimulation. *Vasodepressor* carotid sinus hypersensitivity is a decrease in systolic blood pressure of 50 mm Hg or more without associated cardiac slowing.

ECG Characteristics

Atrial standstill because of sinus arrest or SA exit block coupled with failure of junctional or ventricular escape beats.

Mechanism

Not known. Suspects are excessive resting vagal tone; excessive acetylcholine; hypersensitive baroreflex; inadequate cholinesterase; concomitant sympathetic withdrawal.

Causes

* Coronary artery disease
* Tight collar, head turning, or neck tension (reduces blood flow through the vertebral arteries)

Treatment

Nonsymptomatic patients are not treated. The syndrome may be enhanced by digitalis, alphamethyldopa, clonidine, and propranolol.

Cardioinhibitory form: Generally, atropine and ventricular pacing with or without atrial pacing for symptomatic patients.

Vasodepressor form: Atropine does not prevent a decrease in systemic blood pressure; vasodepression may cause continued syncope even after pacemaker implantation. Elastic support hose and sodium-retaining drugs may be helpful.

PACs and Atrial Tachycardia

7

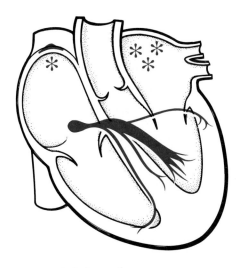

Premature Atrial Complex

A premature atrial complex (PAC) is an atrial impulse that emerges earlier than the next expected sinus beat from a focus other than the sinus node.

ECG Recognition

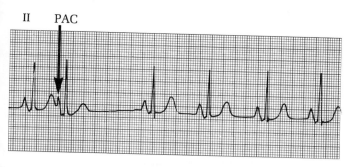

Rate: That of the underlying rhythm.

Rhythm: Irregular, because of the PAC (underlying rhythm may be regular).

P′R interval: The P′-R interval may be the same as the sinus rhythm, or prolonged because of conduction down the slow AV nodal pathway.

QRS complex: Normal or prolonged because of functional or pathological bundle branch block (BBB).

Distinguishing features: The diagnosis is made because of an irregular rhythm and premature P waves that usually have a different shape from that of the sinus P wave. The premature P waves are clearly visible or may distort T waves.

Rhythm Variations

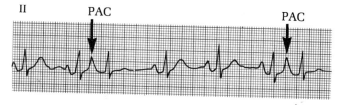

- PACs hidden in T waves. Helpful clues are irregular rhythm (two premature beats); narrow QRS (supraventricular mechanism); and distortion of the Ts preceding the premature beats.

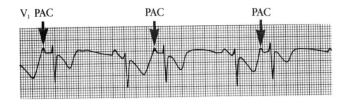

- Bigeminal PACs. Helpful clues are group beating; narrow QRS; and distortion in front of every other beat.

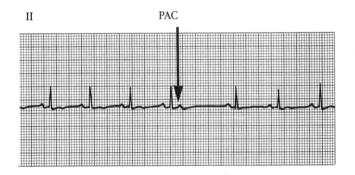

- Nonconducted PAC. Helpful clues are abrupt pause; narrow QRS; and distortion of the T wave preceding the pause.

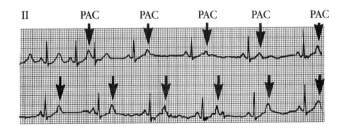

- Bigeminal nonconducted PACs. Helpful clues are sudden, inappropriate, profound bradycardia; narrow QRS; T waves distorted differently each time; and the fact that bigeminal nonconducted PAC is a more common mechanism than SSS.

Mechanism

PACs are the result of abnormal automaticity or triggered activity.

Causes

- Strong emotion (catecholamines)
- Tobacco
- Alcohol
- Caffeine
- Myocardial ischemia
- Infection
- A variety of medications
- Low potassium
- Low magnesium
- Hypoxia
- Stretch of the myocardium (warns of congestive heart failure)
- Dilated or hypertrophied atria because of mitral stenosis or atrial septal defect

▶ Clinical Implications

- May precipitate PSVT, atrial flutter, or atrial fibrillation, and rarely VT.
- In acute MI, PACs are frequently the result of catecholamines released secondary to apprehension and pain or may warn of congestive heart failure and electrolyte imbalance.
- The bradycardia of bigeminal nonconducted PACs may be profound and cause hemodynamic deterioration, even in a healthy heart.

Treatment

PACs themselves are not treated. Look for and treat causes. If they are causing the onset of PSVT, dietary measures may help (more potassium, less caffeine). If they are the result of apprehension and pain (acute MI), reassurance and morphine may cause them to disappear. If they are the result of hypoxia (especially in smokers), oxygen is effective.

Atrial Tachycardia

Atrial tachycardia is the rapid beating of the atria.

ECG Recognition of Nonparoxysmal Atrial Tachycardia

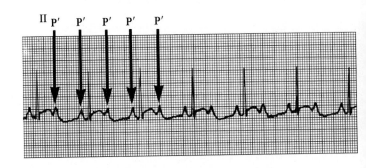

- Digitalis toxic atrial tachycardia

Atrial rate: less than 200 beats/min.

P′ wave: Contour different from that of the sinus P wave, unless the atrial tachycardia is digitalis induced.

P′P′ intervals: Isoelectric line between P′ waves (all leads).

QRS complex: Narrow, unless BBB is also present.

AV conduction: Block is often present (2:1 in example).

Distinguishing features: P′ axis, atrial rate, clinical setting. Rhythm gets faster ("warm up") after onset and slows down before termination ("cool down"), a characteristic common to automaticity.

Effect of vagal maneuvers: No effect except to cause AV block.

ECG Recognition of Paroxysmal Atrial Tachycardia

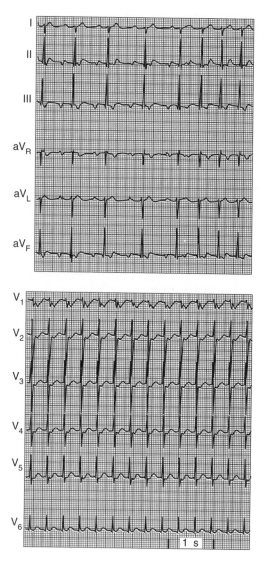

Incessant atrial tachycardia. In the limb leads on the left there is a ratio of 2:1 followed by a ratio 1:1 AV conduction. This patient has been continuously in tachycardia for 12 years and came to medical attention with dilated cardiomyopathy.

From Wellens HJJ. In Willerson JT, Cohn JN: *Cardiovascular medicine,* New York, 1995, Churchill Livingstone.

Atrial rate: 130–180 beats/min.

Rhythm: Usually regular.

P' waves: Polarity determined by the site of the ectopic focus.

P'R interval: Normal or prolonged due to digitalis.

QRS complexes: Normal, unless associated with BBB.

AV conduction: Depends on atrial rate.

Distinguishing features: Paroxysmal; rare (previous atrial surgery, such as for congenital heart disease); may be persistent (present most of the time).

Mechanisms

Nonparoxysmal type: Abnormal automaticity or triggered activity
Paroxysmal type: Reentry (80%); triggered activity

Clinical Implications

- Misdiagnosis; digitalis excess may be mistaken for sinus tachycardia.
- Persistent type results in progressive cardiac dilation and congestive heart failure, which are potentially reversible with ablation of the focus.
- More common when right ventricular dysfunction accompanies inferior wall myocardial infarction.

Pediatrics

Persistent atrial tachycardia is a more common mechanism in children (commonly associated with cardiac tumors or aneurysms) than in adults. As in the adult, the pediatric tachycardia is resistant to medical management. The rate of progression is relatively slow, and the resultant cardiomyopathy is often reversible. His bundle ablation may be necessary to prevent death if medical management fails.

Bedside Diagnosis

- Varying intensity of the first heart sound with varying AV block.
- Excessive number of *a* waves in the jugular venous pulse.
- Carotid sinus massage: Causes increase in AV block and a stepwise slowing of the ventricular rate without termination of the atrial tachycardia. Serious ventricular arrhythmias may result if performed in digitalis toxicity.

Ablation of Atrial Tachycardia

It is possible to ablate the focus for automatic and reentrant atrial tachycardias, the majority of which arise in the crista terminalis (see p. 78). Some are in the left atrium and can be approached with a transseptal technique. Additionally, atrial tachycardias after surgery for congenital heart disease and reentry around a surgical scar, anatomic defect, or atriotomy incision have been successfully ablated.

Treatment of Digitalis Toxicity

Discontinue the drug; avoid sympathetic stimulation; give KC1 intravenously; start phenytoin with a pacing lead in place. Digitalis antibody may be used for symptomatic patients.

Multifocal (Chaotic) Atrial Tachycardia

Multifocal, or chaotic, atrial tachycardia is the rapid firing of atrial ectopic foci from more than two foci.

ECG Recognition

V_1

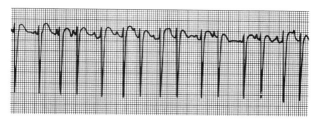

Atrial rate: 100–130 beats/min.
Rhythm: Irregular.
P waves: Three or more different morphologies in a single ECG lead.
PP intervals: Varying; isoelectric PP segment.
PR intervals: Varying.
QRS complexes: Normal unless an intraventricular conduction problem exists.
AV conduction: Usually all P′ waves are conducted to the ventricles.
Distinguishing features: Multiple P′ wave shapes, usually conducted, in patients with chronic obstructive pulmonary disease (COPD).

Mechanism

- Probably triggered activity (responds to calcium channel blockers)
- Proarrhythmic effect of the pathology and treatment of COPD (right atrial enlargement, hypercapnia, hypoxia, and acidosis)

Clinical Implications

- Relatively infrequent
- Usually in critically ill elderly patients
- Often associated with clinically significant pulmonary disease (60%)
- May deteriorate into atrial fibrillation

Pediatrics

In neonates and infants, this arrhythmia is often mistaken for atrial flutter. It is more persistent than atrial flutter, however, and may be associated with atrial septal defect. If drug therapy is successful in slowing the ventricular rate but not that of the atria, the atria dilate, the arrhythmia is exacerbated, and congestive heart failure results.

Treatment

Therapy is directed at correcting the predisposing cardiac, pulmonary, metabolic, and infectious conditions.

Atrial Fibrillation

8

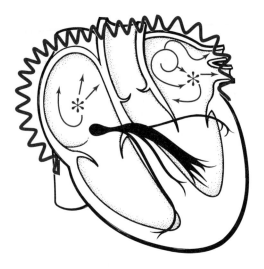

Atrial fibrillation is the disorganized electrical activity of the atria resulting in irregular heartbeat, hemodynamic compromise, risk of thromboembolism, and an increased mortality. It may be acute (onset within 24–48 hours; rapid heart rate); subacute (controlled heart rate); or chronic (paroxysmal, persistent, or permanent). Treatment involves antithrombotic therapy, ventricular rate control, and attempts to convert to normal sinus rhythm. Other designations are as follows.

Lone atrial fibrillation: Absence of any other clinical evidence to suggest a primary cardiac disorder.

Vagally mediated atrial fibrillation: Uncommon form found in middle-aged men; episodes occur during sleep, rest, or postprandially.

Catecholamine-sensitive atrial fibrillation: Found in young women; provoked by stress, exercise, caffeine, or alcohol.

ECG Recognition

V_1

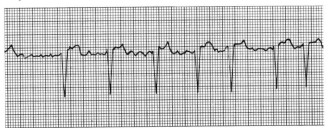

Rate (ventricular): 100–180 beats/min (uncontrolled).

Rhythm: Irregular (intact AV conduction; no surmounting junctional or ventricular rhythm).

P waves: Absent.

QRS complexes: Narrow unless bundle branch block is also present.

Distinguishing features: Absence of P waves and irregular ventricular response (unless AV block or digitalis-toxic, junctional, or fascicular tachycardia)

Other diagnostic features:

- Ventricular rates slower than 100 beats/min suggest AV conduction disease.
- Irregular ventricular rhythm >180 beats/min suggests an accessory pathway (broad QRS) or enhanced AV nodal conduction (narrow QRS).
- Regular ventricular rhythm indicates one of the following:
    1. Conversion to sinus rhythm
    2. Compromised AV conduction (pathological or drug-induced complete AV block)
    3. Drug-induced junctional tachycardia
    4. Drug-induced fascicular ventricular tachycardia (VT)
    5. Conversion to atrial flutter with a fixed conduction ratio

- Group beating indicates one of the following:
  1. Junctional tachycardia with Wenckebach exit block
  2. Fascicular VT (right bundle branch block pattern) with Wenckebach exit block

Rhythm Variations

III

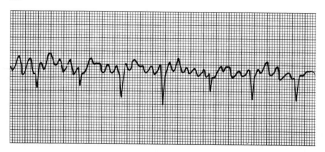

Coarse atrial fibrillation with signs of digitalis toxicity (regularization of the ventricular response). Mortality is 100%. Please see Chapter 17.

II

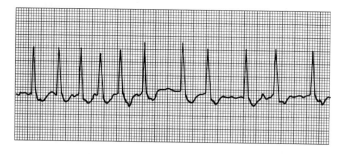

- Fine atrial fibrillation with uncontrolled ventricular response.

V_1

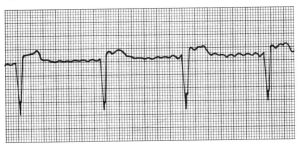

- Atrial fibrillation with complete AV block (note regularity).

II

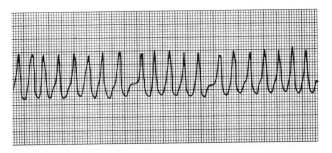

- Atrial fibrillation with conduction over an accessory pathway: broad QRS tachycardia that is irregular and >180 beats/min

Pediatrics

- Rare
- Characterized by rapid ventricular response sometimes exceeding 300 beats/min
- Coarse fibrillatory line on the surface ECG; or fibrillatory line may not be seen
- Usually associated with structurally abnormal heart or Wolff-Parkinson-White (WPW) syndrome

Bedside Diagnosis

- Irregular pulse
- Pulse deficit
- Irregular neck vein pulsation with absence of *a* waves
- Changing systolic blood pressure
- Changing intensity of first heart sound
- Temporary slowing of ventricular rate or no effect from carotid sinus massage
- Awareness of palpitations; hemodynamic collapse, depending on many factors, especially the cardiac status

Physical Assessment

- Check for thromboemboli (peripheral, coronary, pulmonary, or cerebral).
- Look for signs of decreased cardiac output such as hypotension, pulse deficit, signs of heart failure, and decreased cerebral oxygen supply (presyncope or syncope).
- Take pulse by listening for a full minute with stethoscope at the apex.
- In chronic atrial fibrillation, evaluate for digitalis toxicity (QRS regularization or group beating; bradycardia, visual signs, mental signs).
- In chronic atrial fibrillation, evaluate for congestive heart failure (difficulty breathing, pedal edema, crackles at lung bases).

Mechanism

There is a pattern of large macroreentry with transition to very complex patterns of multiple waves of reentry, which collide, becoming wavelets.

Symptoms

- Palpitations
- Varying degrees of hemodynamic compromise, depending on cardiac status
- Polyuria (in paroxysmal atrial fibrillation)
- Exacerbation of angina
- Exercise intolerance

Causes

- Acute myocardial infarction (MI)

- Long-standing hypertension
- Left atrial stretch due to mitral stenosis secondary to rheumatic heart disease or mitral regurgitation
- Postcardiac surgery (30%), especially in the elderly
- Idiopathic or "lone" atrial fibrillation (absence of apparent heart disease)
- Vasodepressor response (vagal)
- Hemodynamic compromise
- Supraventricular tachycardia (SVT)
- Thyrotoxicosis
- Alcohol intake, chronic or acute, moderate to heavy
- Left and right atrial enlargement (cause and consequence)
- Impaired left atrial perfusion (occlusion of the proximal left circumflex artery and the AV nodal artery)
- Pericarditis or heart failure in the first 24 hours of the onset of MI (20% of cases)
- Increased right atrial pressure (inferior and right ventricular MI)
- Increased atrial pressure (acute Q wave anterior MI)

Any type of SVT can overlap with atrial fibrillation.

Clinical Implications

- High risk of thromboembolism (lower in paroxysmal than in chronic form; higher in patients with rheumatic heart disease than without); caused by the inefficient movement of blood in the atria.
- Paroxysmal form more debilitating than the chronic form because of its abrupt onset.
- Mortality depends on the type and severity of underlying heart disease rather than persistence of the arrhythmia.
- Favorable prognosis in lone atrial fibrillation.
- One of the most common symptomatic sustained arrhythmias. Prevalence increases with age.
- Frequently associated with hypertension and structural heart disease.
- Common following cardiac surgery.

Treatment Considerations

- Goals (rate control, anticoagulation, and conversion to sinus rhythm)
- Risks of thromboembolism

Treatment

Acute atrial fibrillation: Rate control or emergency DC synchronized cardioversion.

Paroxysmal atrial fibrillation: Rate control and aspirin.
- Cardioversion is indicated only if rhythm becomes persistent and efforts are going to be made to maintain sinus rhythm afterward.

Persistent and permanent: Rate control, antithrombotic therapy, evaluation of reversible causes (most common are drugs and thyroid disease), consideration of cardioversion.

Atrial Flutter

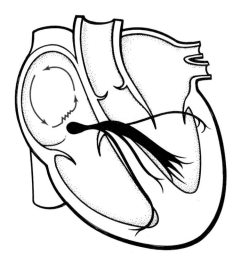

Atrial flutter is a rapid and remarkably regular form of atrial tachycardia that is sustained by a macroreentrant circuit; it is usually paroxysmal, lasting for periods varying from seconds to hours, and occasionally even days.

Flutter-fibrillation is a coarse atrial fibrillation (surface leads) commonly seen as a transitional stage from fibrillation to flutter in patients taking class I antiarrhythmic drugs.

Table 9-1 Types and features of atrial flutter

Type	Mechanism	P' Wave Axis	Atrial Rate	Cure
Typical counterclock-wise (common)	Counterclockwise macroreentry	Superior	240–340 beats/min	RFA[1]
Typical clockwise (rare)	Clockwise macroreentry	Usually inferior; may be superior	240–340 beats/min	RFA
Atypical (rare)	Macroreentry	Inferior	340–433 beats/min	Infrequently RFA
Incisional	Macroreentry	May vary with scar location	Varies	

[1]RFA, Radiofrequency ablation

ECG Findings Common to All Forms of Atrial Flutter

Ventricular rate: Depends on AV conduction ratio; usually 140 to 160 beats/min because of a 2:1 AV conduction ratio.

Ventricular rhythm: Regular if there is a fixed AV conduction ratio; group beating if there is Wenckebach conduction; and irregular if there is variable AV conduction.

Effect of carotid sinus massage: Temporary slowing of the ventricular rate because of AV block, or no effect.

AV conduction ratio: Conduction ratios are usually even (e.g., 2:1, 4:1, 6:1).

Typical Atrial Flutter (Type I)

There are two forms: Counterclockwise rotation of macroreentrant circuit is common; clockwise rotation is rare. Both are seen in patients with or without heart disease and do not require a scar from prior atriotomy. Both can be cured by radiofrequency ablation (RFA).

Counterclockwise Rotation

ECG Recognition

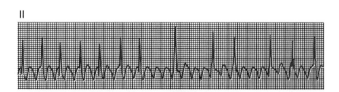

Atrial rate: 240 to 340 beats/min.

Atrial rhythm: Regular.

P′ wave axis: Superior.

Flutter wave: Familiar "sawtooth" appearance. The P′ wave is the negative component of the flutter wave in lead aV$_F$; the Ta wave (atrial repolarization) is positive.

Mechanism

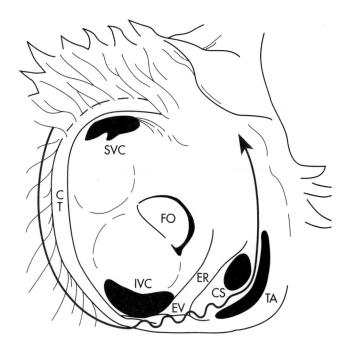

Pertinent atrial structures that form a protected pathway for the macroreentrant circuit are the following:

Crista terminalis: The terminal crest of the right atrium; a ridge on the internal surface of the right atrium located lateral to the orifices of the superior and inferior venae cavae.

Eustachian valve: Valve of the inferior vena cava; it forms its inferior lip.

Eustachian ridge: With the eustachian valve, this ridge forms a barrier to conduction between the inferior vena cava and the coronary sinus.

Coronary sinus: The terminal portion of the great cardiac vein, which empties into the right atrium.

Fossa ovalis: A depression on the right interatrial septum representing the remains of the fetal *foramen ovale*. The fossa ovalis does not participate in the macroreentrant circuit of atrial flutter, but is included here for its landmark value.

Tricuspid annulus: A fibrous ring surrounding the orifice of the tricuspid valve. Barriers to conduction provide a protected pathway for the wave front and prevent stray currents from traversing the smooth-walled posterior right atrium and terminating the mechanism by introducing refractory tissue.

Isthmus of slow conduction: This narrow isthmus of slow conduction can be interrupted by a lesion created by radiofrequency energy, eliminating the possibility of such a reentrant circuit being initiated or sustained, and providing a cure.

Genesis of Flutter Waves

Although atrial flutter is generated by a reentry circuit in the right atrium, the P′ wave polarity on the ECG is determined primarily by the sequence of activation in the left atrium, usually activating it in an inferior/superior direction.

Clinical Implications

- Acute form following open heart surgery; probably caused by the diffuse sterile pericarditis and atrial inflammation associated with the surgical procedure
- May occur during the acute phase of MI
- Associated with pulmonary embolism with or without preexisting cardiac disease
- Chronic form is rare; seen in persons over 40 years of age and is commonly associated with organic heart disease
- High risk if combined with an accessory pathway; ventricular response sometimes 1:1

Pediatrics

- Neonate: Common; atrial rates usually approach 400 beats/min with 2:1 conduction.
- Newborn: Usually associated with normal cardiac structure.
- Treatment: Transesophageal overdrive pacing or external synchronized cardioversion. Once treated, in some it may never return. Most infants outgrow this arrhythmia by 12 to 18 months of age.

Bedside Diagnosis

- Rapid, rippling flutter waves seen in the jugular venous pulse if AV conduction is 4:1.

- First heart sound has a constant intensity if the AV relationship remains constant.
- You may hear the rapid sounds of the atrial contractions if AV conduction is 4:1.
- The pulse is regular if the conduction ratio is fixed.

Acute Treatment

- Depends on the clinical setting
- DC cardioversion (<50 joules) or rapid atrial pacing
- Antiarrhythmic drug therapy may be initiated prior to either DC cardioversion or pacing. Following are the goals of drug therapy:
  1. Slow the ventricular rate.
  2. Restore sinus rhythm.
  3. Enhance the effect of rapid atrial pacing.
  4. Maintain sinus rhythm once converted.

Long-Term Treatment—A Cure

Radiofrequency catheter ablation to create persistent bidirectional conduction block in the inferior vena cava–tricuspid annulus isthmus.

Clockwise Rotation

ECG Recognition

Atrial rate: 240 to 340 beats/min.
Atrial rhythm: Regular.
P′ wave axis: Usually inferior, but may be superior.
Flutter wave: The P′ wave portion of the flutter wave is usually positive (and negative Ta wave) in inferior leads caused by the inferior P′ axis. However, the P′ axis may be superior with flutter waves identical to those of the more common counterclockwise form of atrial flutter. The P′ waves in V_1 may have an undulating diphasic pattern or may mimic the positive P′ wave of the more common counterclockwise mechanism.

Mechanism

The clockwise macroreentry route is anatomically identical to that of the counterclockwise rotation.

Acute Treatment

Same as for counterclockwise typical atrial flutter.

Atypical Atrial Flutter (Type II)

A rare form of rapid macroreentrant atrial tachycardia.

ECG Recognition

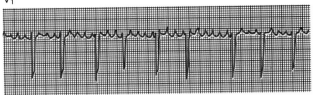

Atrial rate: 340 to 433 beats/min.
Atrial rhythm: Regular.
P′ wave axis: Inferior.
Flutter wave: The P′ component of the flutter wave is positive in the inferior leads, similar to the clockwise form of typical atrial flutter; the P′ in the precordial leads is also positive.

Mechanism

Not yet known.

Genesis of Flutter Waves

The positive component of the F wave (the P′) reflects the descending limb of the reentry circuit in the intraatrial septum and left atrium, the chamber that determines the morphology of the P′ wave. The ascending limb is not reflected on the surface ECG.

Treatment

Atypical atrial flutter is difficult to terminate, and radiofrequency ablation is difficult to achieve.

Incisional Reentrant Atrial Tachycardia

Complication in 25% of patients following repair of complex congenital heart disease. Although classified as atrial flutter, it differs significantly from typical atrial flutter.

Mechanism

An essential electrophysiological substrate is an isthmus of myocardium between the atriotomy scar and the atriopulmonary connection.

Long-Term Treatment

Ablated with good success rate using focused activation mapping and radiofrequency ablation to transect a critical isthmus of conductive tissue between two nonconductive regions.

Junctional Beats and Rhythms

10

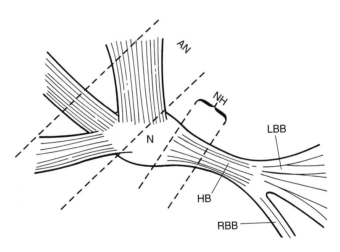

The divisions of the AV junction. *AN,* Atrionodal; *N,* compact AV node; *NH,* nodal-His; *HB,* His bundle; *LBB,* left bundle branch; *RBB,* right bundle branch.

Terminology

Nonparoxysmal: Of gradual onset and termination.

Accelerated Junctional Rhythm: A junctional rate of more than 60 and less than 100 beats/min.

Junctional Tachycardia: Strict sense: a junctional rate of 100 beats/min or more; functional sense: a junctional rate of greater than its normal escape rate.

Accelerated Idiojunctional Rhythm: Independent beating of the AV junction.

Retrograde Conduction: Conduction up the AV node or an accessory pathway.

AV Dissociation: The independent beating of atria and ventricles.

AV Junction: The AV node and bundle of His to its branching portion.

AN Region: A transitional zone of gradually merging atrial and compact AV nodal fibers.

The N Region: The compact AV node, especially the midnodal region.

The NH Region: A transitional zone of merging lower AV nodal and His bundle fibers.

Premature Junctional Complex

A premature junctional complex (PJC) originates in the AV junction. It discharges before the next expected sinus impulse and activates the ventricles through the His bundle and bundle branches in the normal manner (narrow QRS).

ECG Recognition

Rate: That of the underlying rhythm.

Rhythm: Irregular because of the PJC.

P′ wave: If a P′ wave occurs, it is negative in leads II, III, and aVF and may be before, during, or after the QRS.

P′R interval: If the P′ wave occurs before the QRS, the P′R interval is less than 0.12 sec.

QRS complex: Normal in shape and duration unless there is an intraventricular conduction abnormality.

Distinguishing features: A premature narrow QRS with no associated P wave or retrograde P′ wave immediately before, during, or after the QRS.

Examples of PJCs

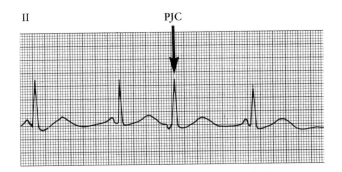

- PJC with the P′ preceding the QRS complex.

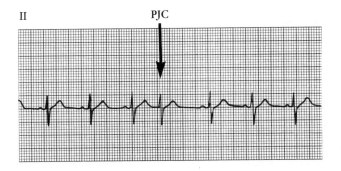

- PJC with the P′ hidden in the QRS complex; the sinus node is reset with this beat.

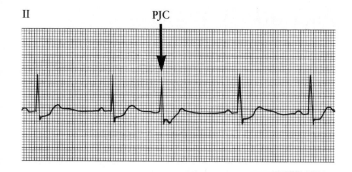

II   PJC

- PJC with the P′ following the QRS complex.

Causes

- Ischemia or hypoxia
- Digitalis
- Acute inferior wall MI
- Tricuspid prosthesis
- Rheumatic fever

Treatment

None.

Nonparoxysmal Junctional Tachycardia

Nonparoxysmal junctional tachycardia is a narrow QRS tachycardia with gradual onset and termination that originates within AV junctional fibers (AV node/His bundle).

ECG Recognition

Rate: The rate is 70 to 140 beats/min (may emerge at 60–70 beats/min if there is sinus bradycardia or SA block). In patients receiving digitalis, junctional rate gradually increases as more digitalis is given.

Rhythm: Nonparoxysmal; may slowly increase its rate.

P waves: Retrograde P′ waves before, during, or after the QRS. If there is AV dissociation, the atrial rhythm may be normal sinus, atrial fibrillation, atrial tachycardia, or atrial flutter.

P′R interval: Less than 0.12 sec if the P′ wave occurs before the QRS.

QRS complex: Normal in duration and shape unless there is an intraventricular conduction abnormality.

Response to carotid sinus massage: None.

Examples of Junctional Tachycardia

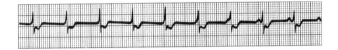

- Junctional tachycardia from a suicide attempt with digitalis; the atrial rate and the junctional rate are similar (isorhythmic AV dissociation).

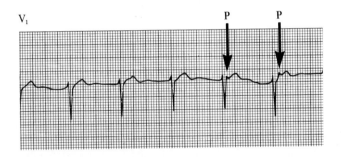

- Accelerated idiojunctional rhythm.

Mechanism

Enhanced normal automaticity, abnormal automaticity, or triggered activity.

Causes

- Digitalis toxicity
- Inferior MI
- Myocarditis, often secondary to acute rheumatic fever

- Post–open heart surgery
- Idiopathic

Pediatrics

Postoperative junctional tachycardia often occurs in infants following complex open heart surgery; it abates after 48 to 72 hours. The rate is responsive to temperature, catecholamines, and decreased vagal tone and can be controlled by cooling, electrolyte replacement, enhancement of vagal tone, and reduction in sympathetic stimulation. If medical management fails, His bundle ablation may be life saving. In congenital nonparoxysmal junctional tachycardia, the infant mortality is relatively high.

Physical Signs

- Nonparoxysmal junctional tachycardia is determined by ventricular rate, atrial rate, P-QRS relationship (atrial kick), ventricular function, and underlying heart disease.
- The first heart sound varies in intensity if AV dissociation is present; it is of constant intensity if AV dissociation is not present.
- Irregular cannon *a* waves are present in jugular pulse if AV dissociation is present.

Treatment

Usually none. If there is digitalis toxicity, it is usually sufficient to discontinue the drug. If there is hemodynamic compromise, digitalis antibody may be life saving.

Junctional Escape Beats and Rhythms

Junctional escape beats and rhythms are impulses discharged from the AV junction when the sinus node is too slow or fails.

ECG Recognition

Heart rate: Bradycardia (35–60 beats/min; junctional escape rhythm).

Rhythm: Irregular for junctional escape beats and regular for junctional escape rhythms.

QRS complex: Normal or the same shape as the sinus conducted beats.

Distinguishing features: Underlying bradycardia or pauses that are terminated by the appearance of a normal QRS with or without a retrograde P′.

Rhythm Variations

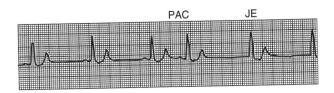

- Junctional escape (JE) terminates the pause after the PAC.

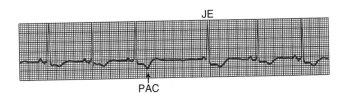

- JE beat follows a pause created by a nonconducted PAC. The sinus P wave in front of the JE beat is too close to have been conducted.

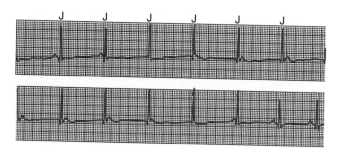

Sinus bradycardia with a junctional escape rhythm of 58 beats/min, resulting in AV dissociation (continuous tracing). If you mark off the first two P waves, they can be "walked out" through the tracing when they distort the QRS in front and in back or are completely hidden within the QRS. The first P wave in the tracing may conduct to the ventricles. (The PR interval is 0.12 sec.) Because the RR intervals are exactly the same across the tracing, the first QRS is probably a junctional beat as well.

- Sinus bradycardia with a junctional escape rhythm (J) of 58 beats/min.

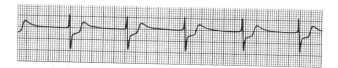

- Junctional escape rhythm of 60 beats/min.

Mechanism

The inherent rate of junctional cells is 35 to 60 beats/min. They may pace the heart when the sinus node defaults (e.g., marked sinus bradycardia, SA block, during the pause caused by a nonconducted PAC, or AV block).

Treatment

Usually none.

Paroxysmal Supraventricular Tachycardia

11

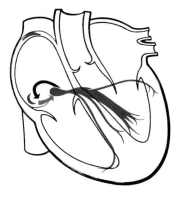

AV nodal reentry
tachycardia

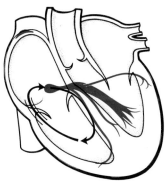

Circus movement
tachycardia
(AV reciprocating)

The two most common mechanisms of paroxysmal supraventricular tachycardia (PSVT) are AV nodal reentry tachycardia (AVNRT) and orthodromic circus movement tachycardia (CMT). Other mechanisms are SA nodal reentry (p. 54), antidromic CMT, and rarely atrial tachycardia (p. 63).

Emergency Response to PSVT

Emergency treatment for AVNRT and CMT is exactly the same; long-term treatment differs slightly.

Hemodynamically Stable Patient

- **Record** the tachycardia in at least 5 leads (I, II, III, V_1, V_6).
- **Terminate** the tachycardia.[1]
    1. Use the vagal maneuver. If unsuccessful, proceed with step 2.
    2. Give adenosine 6 mg IV rapidly; if unsuccessful, increase the dosage to 12 mg; this may be repeated once. If unsuccessful, go to step 3.
    3. Give procainamide hydrochloride 10 mg/kg body weight IV over 5 minutes. If unsuccessful, go to step 4.
    4. Use electrical cardioversion.
- **Record** the sinus rhythm in the same leads.
- **Stabilize** the patient and take a history.
- **Diagnose** by close examination of the tracings with and without the tachycardia.
- **Refer** the patient for radiofrequency ablation if CMT or refractory AVNRT are diagnosed.

Hemodynamically Unstable Patient

- **Record** the rhythm in at least 5 leads.
- **Terminate** with synchronized D.C. cardioversion.
- **Record** the sinus rhythm in the same leads.
- **Stabilize** the patient, and take a history.
- **Diagnose** by close examination of the tracings with and without the tachycardia.
- **Refer** for radiofrequency ablation if CMT or refractory AVNRT are diagnosed.

---

[1]Wellens HJJ, Conover M: *The ECG in emergency decision making,* Philadelphia, 1992, WB Saunders.

AV Nodal Reentry Tachycardia

ECG Recognition

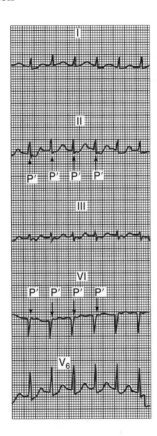

The pseudo-S waves in II, III, and V_6, and the pseudo r waves in V_1, are the P' waves peeking out of the QRS.

Heart rate: 170 to 250 beats/min.

Rhythm: Regular or irregular (varying AV nodal conduction).

Initiating P'R interval: Approximately 0.38 sec (slow pathway conduction time).

Location of the P' waves: Buried within the QRS and not seen at all, or distorting the end of the QRS.

Polarity of the P′ waves: Negative in leads II, III, and aV_F; positive in lead V_1.

QRS complex: Narrow, but often distorted by the P′ wave, causing a pseudo S wave in the inferior leads, a pseudo r′ in lead V_1, or both.

Conduction ratio: 1 : 1.

Aberrant ventricular conduction: Uncommon.

Distinguishing features: Recognized immediately as a paroxysmal, narrow QRS tachycardia (aberrancy is rare). Close examination often reveals pseudo s waves in inferior leads, pseudo r′ waves in V_1, or both. If the initiating PAC is seen, the P′R interval will be long.

Mechanism

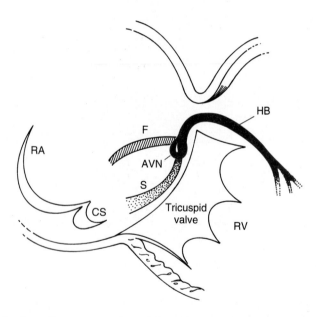

A schematic representation of the right atrium (RA) and right ventricle (RV) opened to reveal the compact atrioventricular node (AVN) and its atrial fibers. The fast fibers are superior; the slow fibers are inferior, arising near the os of the coronary sinus (CS).

Adapted from Kiem S, Werner P, Jazayeri M et al: Circulation, 86:919, 1992.

- AVNRT is possible because of two functionally separate pathways (slow and fast) running along opposite edges of the compact AV node into the right atrium in a fanlike fashion.

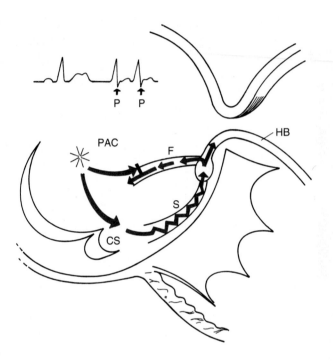

- The refractory period of the slow pathway is the shortest; therefore, when a PAC arrives at the approaches to the AV node, it may be conducted only down the slow pathway. Within the AV node it travels in two directions: up the fast pathway to the atrium (a reciprocal beat) and down the His bundle to the ventricles.

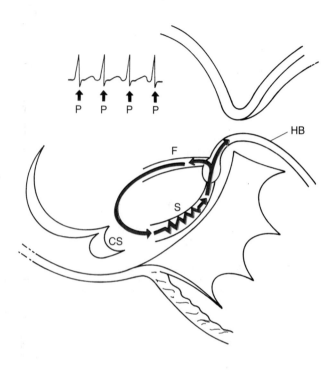

- A reentry circuit is thus established. The atria and ventricles are activated simultaneously, placing the P′ wave within the QRS.

Clinical Implications

- Usually benign and self-limiting
- Easily terminated by a vagal maneuver
- Occasionally refractory to treatment and referred for radiofrequency ablation

Bedside Diagnosis

- Regular pulse
- "Frog sign" (regular cannon 'a' waves in the jugular venous pulse; identifies PSVT but does not differentiate between AVNRT and CMT)
- Constant systolic blood pressure

- Constant intensity of first heart sound
- Carotid sinus massage may terminate PSVT or may have no effect

Long-Term Treatment (Cure)

Transvenous radiofrequency ablation.

Orthodromic CMT (Rapidly Conducting Accessory Pathway)

ECG Recognition

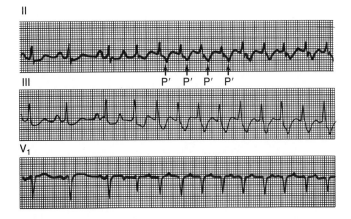

The P′ waves are easily seen in V_1 and follow the QRS in leads II and III.

Heart rate: 170 to 250 beats/min.

Rhythm: Regular, but may be irregular owing to changing conduction through the AV node.

Initiating P′R interval: Not prolonged.

Location of the P′ waves: Always separate from the QRS.

Polarity of the P′ waves: Depends on the atrial insertion of the accessory pathway.

Left atrial insertion: Lead I, negative P′; lead II and III, equiphasic or positive.

Right atrial insertion: Lead I, positive P′; lead II, equiphasic or positive; lead III, negative.

Posteroseptal insertion: Leads II and III, negative P′.

QRS complex: Normal unless there is aberrant ventricular conduction.

Conduction ratio: Always 1:1.

Aberrant ventricular conduction: Common.

Heart rate during aberrancy: Slower than without aberrancy if the accessory pathway is on the same side as the BBB.

QRS alternans: Common.

Distinguishing features: Like AVNRT, CMT is recognized immediately as a PSVT, although aberrancy is common. Unlike CMT, close examination reveals separate P′ waves that closely follow the QRS. If the initiating PAC is seen, the P′R interval is not prolonged.

Rhythm Variations

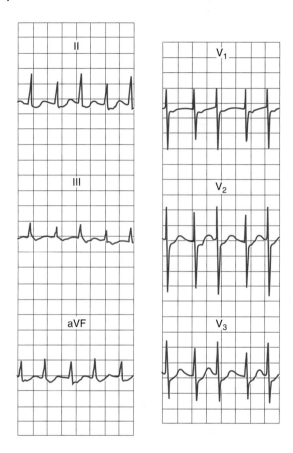

- QRS alternans during CMT helps to locate the P′ following the QRS.

V₁

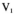

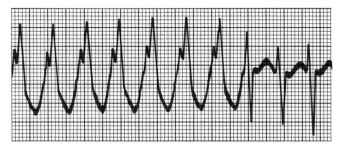

- CMT with RBBB aberrancy. Note that the heart rate during aberrancy is slower than it is without aberrancy. The blocked right bundle forces the reentry current to pass first down the left bundle, a longer route to this right-sided accessory pathway.

Mechanism: AV Reentry

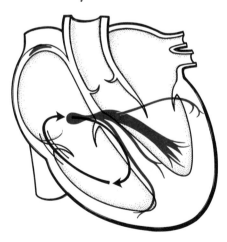

Note that there are two AV pathways providing a pathway for the reentry loop: (1) the AV node and His bundle (anterograde conduction) and (2) an accessory pathway (retrograde conduction). Commonly a PAC, or less commonly a PVC, initiates the tachycardia.

Initiation With a PAC

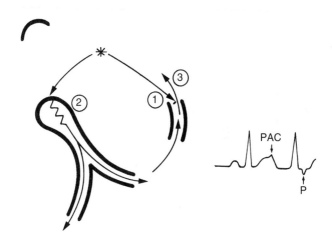

1. A PAC is blocked in the accessory pathway.
2. The impulse passes down the AV node into the ventricles.
3. The impulse returns quickly to the atria via the accessory pathway.

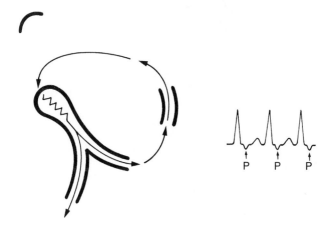

A reentry circuit is established (AV node-ventricles-accessory pathway-atria, in sequence); note P′ wave separate from QRS.

Causes

Presence of an accessory pathway, and a critically timed PAC or PVC or an accelerated sinus rhythm in the young.

Clinical Implications

- Orthodromic CMT may lead to atrial fibrillation with heart rates greater than 200 beats/min, which may precipitate ventricular fibrillation.
- A cure is available at centers skilled in the use of radiofrequency ablation.

Bedside Diagnosis

Same as for AVNRT.

Long-Term Treatment (Cure)

After the resolution of the acute event, the patient should be referred to a center experienced in the treatment of the arrhythmias or WPW syndrome. A cure is available in the form of radiofrequency ablation.

Orthodromic CMT (Slowly Conducting Accessory Pathway)

ECG Recognition

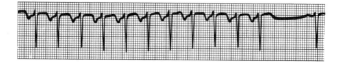

Note the long R-P′ interval because of the slowly conducting accessory pathway.

Rhythm: Described as "incessant," "persistent," "permanent." Although respite from this rhythm is seldom, its onset is paroxysmal, often beginning after a sinus cycle.

QRS complex: Narrow.

P′ location: RP interval greater than PR interval.

P′ polarity: Negative in II, III, and aVF.

Distinguishing features: Easily recognized because the RP interval is greater than the P′R interval; the rhythm occupies more than 12 hours/day and causes congestive heart failure. Looks like a junctional tachycardia because of the negative P' waves in the inferior leads.

Mechanism

The reentry circuit consists of conduction into the ventricles via the AV node (narrow QRS) and retrograde conduction to the atria via a slowly conducting accessory pathway, placing the P' wave well beyond the QRS (RP > PR).

Clinical Implications

Atrial damage and congestive heart failure result from the many hours/day in SVT. Although this form of CMT is very rare, it is extremely important to recognize it, because a complete cure is available.

Treatment

Radiofrequency ablation of the accessory pathway is a cure. The tachycardia-related cardiomyopathy then resolves considerably.

Antidromic CMT

Antidromic CMT is a rare form of PSVT.

ECG Recognition

Rate: Greater than 170 beats/min.
Rhythm: Regular.
QRS complex: Identical to VT with a focus at the base of the ventricles.
Distinguishing features: Broad QRS tachycardia identical in form to VT.

Mechanism

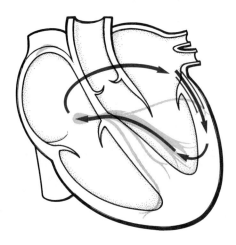

The reentry circuit uses the accessory pathway anterogradely and the His bundle and AV node retrogradely, producing a tachycardia identical in appearance to VT with a basal focus.

Causes

- A critically timed PAC or PVC
- Presence of an accessory pathway

▶ Clinical Implications

Patients with antidromic CMT often (50%) have multiple accessory pathways and should be referred to centers skilled in the use of radiofrequency ablation techniques. Definitive diagnosis can only be made with electrophysiological studies.

Emergency and Long-Term Treatment

Same as for orthodromic CMT.

Table 11-1   ECG differential diagnosis in PSVT

ECG Sign	AVNRT	CMT
QRS alternans	Rare	Common
Initial P'R	Prolonged	Normal
P' wave location	Hidden in the QRS or may look like terminal QRS forces	Separate from QRS (always)
P' polarity	Negative in inferior leads (pseudo s wave); positive in lead V_1 (pseudo r')	Varies with accessory pathway location
Aberrancy	Rare	Common
Heart rate during aberrancy	Same as without aberrancy	May be slower than without aberrancy
AV conduction	Usually 1:1	Always 1:1

Physical Signs of PSVT

- Irregular pulse
- BP constant
- Constant intensity of S_1
- "Frog sign" (rapid, regular expansion of the neck veins)

Pediatrics: PSVT in the Fetus and Neonate

CMT is the most common arrhythmia in the neonate and accounts for most of the PSVTs that occur in infants.

ECG Recognition

Heart rate: 300 beats/min.

Mechanisms in fetus: Intraatrial reentry and atrioventricular reentry.

Diagnosis: Noted during random fetal heart rate monitoring or with fetal sonogram; rarely, the mother will report a decrease in fetal movements.

Treatment

Half of the children with PSVT will be asymptomatic after their first year. The PSVT usually returns by the time they are 20 years of age. Until then, no treatment is required.

▶ Clinical Implications

A rate of 300 beats/min is well tolerated in an infant up to 1 year. In the fetus, a rate of 300 beats/min results in hydrops fetalis in just a few hours.

Carotid Sinus Massage

This strong vagal maneuver is performed by the physician in the hospital setting.

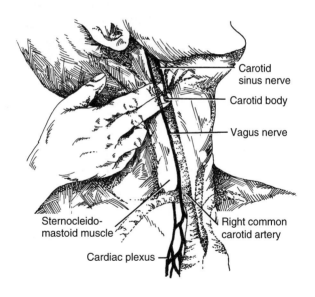

The carotid sinus (carotid body) is located at the bifurcation of the carotid artery at the angle of the jaw. Begin with slight pressure to test for hypersensitivity. Then press the carotid sinus against the lateral processes of the cervical vertebrae with a massaging action for 5 sec.
Caution: do not use on patients >65 years of age.

Premature Ventricular Complexes

12

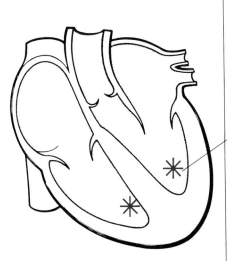

PVC

Ventricular tachycardia

Ventricular fibrillation

Torsades de pointes

Accelerated idioventricular rhythm

Ventricular parasystole

Ventricular fusion

Ventricular flutter

Ventricular escape

A premature ventricular complex (PVC) or ventricular premature beat (VPB) is a single beat or a pair of ventricular ectopic beats that occurs before the expected sinus-conducted QRS.

ECG Recognition

V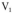

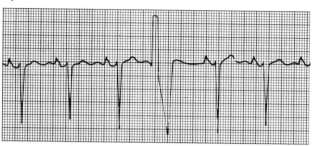

Heart rate: Normal or abnormal.

Rhythm: Irregular due to the PVC.

P wave: Not related to the PVC unless there is retrograde conduction.

PP intervals: Can be "walked out" across the PVC 50% of the time.

QRS complex of the PVC: Broad, premature, increased amplitude.

Full compensatory pause: Present 50% of the time.

T wave of the PVC: Opposite in polarity to the terminal QRS.

Distinguishing features: Easily recognized because it is premature and broad with no related P wave, increased amplitude, and a T wave of opposite polarity to the terminal QRS.

Mechanisms

- Enhanced normal automaticity in the His-Purkinje system (catecholamines)
- Abnormal automaticity anywhere in the ventricles (ischemia, electrolyte imbalance, injury)
- Reentry through slowly conducting tissue within the ventricles (ischemia or injury)
- Triggered activity occurring within the His-Purkinje system (digitalis excess or catecholamines) or within the ventricular myocardium (class IA or IC drugs, for example)

Broad QRS: Widths of > 0.14 sec occur because activation begins outside of the conduction system. Exceptions are fascicular ventricular beats (Chapter 17) and fusion beats (Chapter 23). PVCs may also appear to be narrow in certain leads when initial or terminal forces are isoelectric.

QRS shape: If V_1 is positive, a PVC is monophasic, is biphasic, or has two peaks with the initial peak highest (rabbit ear sign). If V_1 is negative, a PVC has any one of the following: R wave broader than 0.03 sec, a slurred S downstroke, delayed S nadir in V_1 or V_2, or q in V_6.

Increased amplitude: The sequence of activation is such that most currents are traveling in one direction without the canceling-out effect of the normal activation sequence. The resultant vector is stronger.

T wave of opposite polarity: Whenever the process of depolarization is abnormal, the repolarization sequence will produce a T wave that is opposite in polarity to the terminal part of the QRS (secondary T wave change).

The full compensatory pause: A full compensatory pause follows a PVC and is caused by nonconduction of a normal sinus beat.

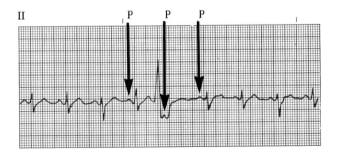

In the tracing above, note that the sinus P wave can be seen in the T wave of the PVC and that the sinus rhythm is undisturbed, causing the next P wave to be on time. This sequence is what is measured when looking for a full compensatory pause. It is possible to have a PVC with less than or more than a full compensatory pause because of sinus arrhythmia or retrograde conduction to the atria. Early discharge of the atria (retrograde conduction) may also cause the pause to be more than "compensatory" because of *overdrive suppression,* a property belonging to all pacemaker cells by which their premature discharge causes their cycle to lengthen.

Types of PVCs

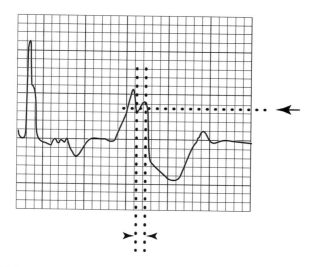

Moulton KP, Medcalf T, Lazzara R: *Circulation* 81:1245, 1990.

The "ugly" PVC[1] is broad (>0.16 sec) with a notch of > 0.04 sec, indicating a dilated and globally hypokinetic left ventricle in a nonspecifically diseased heart. The smooth narrower PVC, on the other hand, reflects normal heart size and normal or near-normal systolic function despite the presence of underlying disease. One measures ugliness (i.e., the notch) by drawing a horizontal line at the level of the lowest point in the notch and making vertical lines at the two peaks.

---

[1]Moulton KP, Medcalf T, and Lazzara R: Premature ventricular complex morphology, a marker for left ventricular structure and function, *Circulation* 81:1245–1251, 1990.

Unifocal and Multifocal

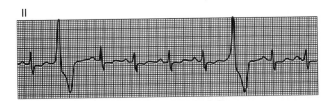

- Unifocal PVCs originate in the same focus, take the same route of conduction, and have identical shapes.

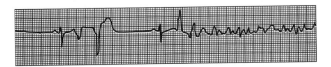

Multifocal or multiform PVCs have different foci. These PVCs are occurring on the T wave in a patient with ischemic heart disease and result in ventricular fibrillation.

- Multifocal PVCs produce a bigeminal rhythm in a patient with atrial fibrillation and digitalis toxicity.

Bigeminy, Trigeminy, Quadrigeminy, and Pairs

II

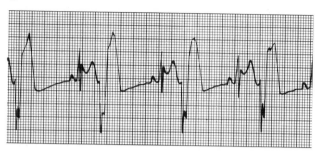

- Ventricular bigeminy. Note the precise coupling of every sinus beat to a PVC; this is commonly seen in coronary artery disease (reentry) and in digitalis toxicity (triggered activity).

V_1

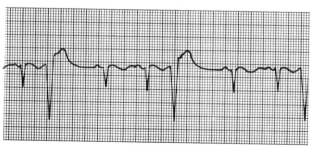

- Ventricular trigeminy (two normal and one PVC).

II

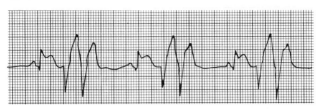

- Ventricular trigeminy (one normal and two PVCs).

V_1

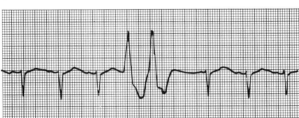

- Paired, or "back-to-back," PVCs that are unifocal.

End-Diastolic PVCs

II

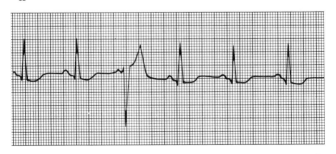

End-diastolic PVC occurs late in the cardiac cycle before the ventricles can be activated or partially activated by the sinus beat; it is often a fusion beat.

Interpolated PVCs

II

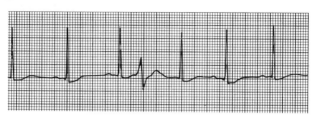

The interpolated PVC is sandwiched between two normal sinus-conducted beats, so it does not have a full compensatory pause.

Fascicular PVCs

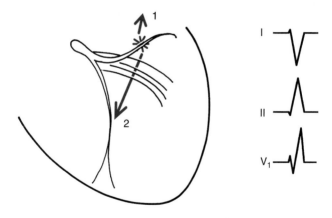

An anterior fascicular beat and its ECG complexes. The QRS is relatively narrow (< 0.14 sec) because of an origin within the conduction system. There is right axis deviation and a right bundle branch block pattern. The indicated 1-2 conduction sequence explains the right axis deviation and the QRS shape in the limb leads.

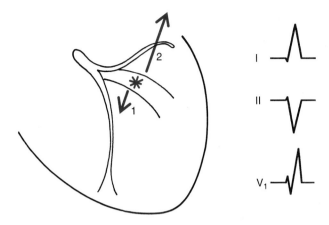

A posterior fascicular beat and its ECG complexes. The QRS is relatively narrow (< 0.14 sec) because of an origin within the conduction system. There is left axis deviation and a right bundle branch block pattern. The indicated 1-2 conduction sequence explains the left axis deviation and the QRS shape in the limb leads.

Ectopic beats originating in the fascicles are < 0.14 sec and look like RBBB aberration. Anterior fascicular beats have right axis deviation, and posterior fascicular beats have left axis deviation. They are seen in digitalis toxicity (Chapter 17).

R-on-T Phenomenon

II

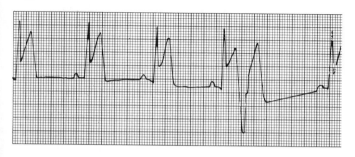

The term *R-on-T* is used to indicate that an R wave (PVC) has occurred at the peak of the T wave—the vulnerable period of the ECG. During the first 4 hours following the onset of symptoms of MI, primary VF and R-on-T ventricular ectopic beats are frequent. They decrease rapidly with time but are clearly a cause for concern when it appears in adults with a history of ischemic heart disease. The mechanism is thought to be the early afterdepolarizations.

Rule of Bigeminy

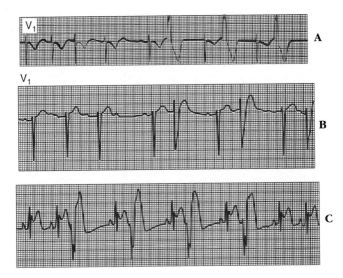

A long cycle tends to precipitate a PVC after the next supraventricular beat.[1] The long cycle in this tracing is produced by AV Wenckebach; when the P wave is not conducted, there is a pause, and ventricular bigeminy results.

Clinical Implications

- A common occurrence, even without heart disease
- Increase in number with age
- Greater risk with acute myocardial infarction
- Aggravated by ischemia, increased sympathetic activity, and increased or reduced heart rate

Other causes include fever, volume depletion, infection, drug excesses of all types, hypokalemia, hypercalcemia, and excess or even moderate alcohol intake in certain individuals.

[1]Langendorf R, Pick A, Winternitz M: Mechanisms of intermittent bigeminy. 1. Appearance of ectopic beats dependent upon the length of the ventricular cycle, the "rule of bigeminy," *Circulation* 11:422, 1955.

Pediatrics

PVCs may occur in children (especially pubertal or prepubertal) with no detectable heart disease. These PVCs are considered benign.

Treatment

None as long as the patient remains asymptomatic.

Monomorphic Ventricular Tachycardia

13

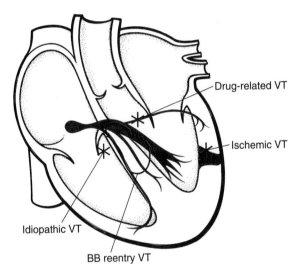

Drug-related VT

Ischemic VT

Idiopathic VT

BB reentry VT

Monomorphic VT is regular with uniform beat-to-beat morphology; it can be sustained, nonsustained, idiopathic, or caused by bundle branch reentry.

ECG Recognition

V_1

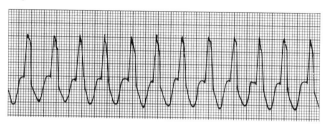

Heart rate: 100 beats/min or more.
Rhythm: Regular.
P waves: Dissociated or retrograde.
QRS complex: Broad.
Distinguishing features:

- AV dissociation or retrograde P′ waves
- Uniform beat-to-beat appearance

Diagnosis

- Evaluate QRS morphology in light of information from the history and physical.
- Be aware that some monomorphic VTs look like SVT with aberration (idiopathic VT, bundle branch reentry VT, and fascicular VT) and that some SVTs look like VT (when there is an accessory pathway).

Other noninvasive tests:

1. A 24-hour ambulatory recording or event recording
2. Provocation of the tachycardia with exercise testing
3. The upright tilt test
4. Signal averaged ECG (risk stratification in MI)
5. Echocardiography, thallium exercise testing, or testing for ejection fraction
6. Electrophysiologic study with programmed stimulation (when symptoms are thought to be caused by arrhythmias, but the physician is unable to diagnose or treat them)

Mechanisms (See Also Chapter 5)

- Reentry. Most instances of chronic sustained VT associated with coronary artery disease, MI, and dilated cardiomyopathy arise as a result of reentry.
- Abnormal automaticity. Ischemia causes abnormal automaticity and slow conduction.
- Triggered activity (digitalis intoxication or excessive catecholamines).

Incidence

- Early phase (first 4 hours after the onset of chest pain): All types of ventricular arrhythmias are frequent, including primary ventricular fibrillation (VF) and R-on-T phenomenon, the incidence of which decreases rapidly with time.
- Late phase: The incidence of VT and PVCs (back-to-back and isolated) increases.

Clinical Implications

Nonsustained ventricular tachycardia: Definitely a risk factor for sudden cardiac death in post-MI patients. When episodes are frequent, rapid, prolonged, and occur in the second week after anterior infarction, they may be warning signs of VF.

Sustained ventricular tachycardia: Commonly seen in adults with prior MI, chronic coronary artery disease, or dilated cardiomyopathy and in those with no apparent structural heart disease (idiopathic VT).

Emergency Treatment

- Management of sustained broad QRS tachycardia with hemodynamic decompensation:
  1. Obtain a 12-lead ECG.
  2. Promptly begin DC cardioversion; very low energies can terminate VT. Begin with a synchronized shock of 10 to 50 watt-seconds.
  3. Digitalis-induced VT: Fab fragments (Digibind).
  4. Obtain a history.
  5. Examine pre- and post-cardioversion ECGs to determine mechanism.

- Management of sustained broad QRS tachycardia without hemo-dynamic decompensation:
  1. Evaluate 12-lead ECG to confirm the diagnosis.
  2. Look for signs of AV dissociation.
  3. Obtain a history.
  4. Start IV procainamide hydrochloride, 6 to 13 mg/kg, at 0.2 to 0.5 mg/kg/min (14–35 mg/min).
  5. If unsuccessful, begin DC cardioversion (synchronized 10 to 50 watt-seconds).
- When in doubt, do not give verapamil; give procainamide hydrochloride.
- Looks like VT, irregular, and >180 beats/min:
  1. Give procainamide; do not give verapamil or digitalis (atrial fibrillation with conduction over an accessory pathway is highly suspect).
- If SVT with aberrancy is suspected in a stable patient:
  1. Try a vagal maneuver (carotid sinus massage or Valsalva).
  2. If unsuccessful, use adenosine. The effect is transient and should not make VT worse.

Differential Diagnosis

- Older patients:
  1. Evaluate for coronary artery disease.
  2. Assess biventricular function.
  3. Evaluate for BB reentry during electrophysiological study.
- Younger patients (without overt heart disease or with isolated right ventricular disease):
  1. Do a noninvasive evaluation of ventricular sizes and function.
  2. An abnormal SAECG (Chapter 25) or identification of intracardiac late potentials suggests right ventricular dysplasia or cardiomyopathy.
  3. Adenosine response and absence of detectable heart disease support a diagnosis of idiopathic right VT.
  Note: Consider right-sided or septal accessory pathways.

Idiopathic VT

Most patients with VT but without structural heart disease have an excellent prognosis. Sudden cardiac death is rare as opposed to the very high mortality associated with postischemic recurrent VT. Frequent episodes of this arrhythmia may result in cardiomyopathy and would render the decision for radiofrequency ablation of the focus more imperative.

Pediatric Prognosis and Treatment

Arrhythmia often disappears; prognosis is favorable. However, treatment and follow-up are required for sustained, symptomatic, or very rapid VT. Radiofrequency catheter ablation is safe and effective treatment for right ventricular outflow tachycardia during childhood and adolescence. However, late effects are unknown.

Most Common Origin of VT in Children

Under 5 years: Hamartoma[1]
Older: Surgery
Other: Long QT syndrome, myocarditis, cardiomyopathy, arrhythmogenic right ventricular dysplasia, coronary artery anomalies

Emergency Treatment

Manage this like other VTs. Verapamil is contraindicated for all wide QRS tachycardias unless the physician is an expert electrophysiologist. Adenosine can be used and is effective for some of the right ventricular outflow tract VTs.

Long-Term Treatment

Radiofrequency ablation is a cure; symptomatic patients are treated, especially if their tachycardia has resulted in cardiomyopathy.

Idiopathic Right Ventricular Tachycardia

ECG recognition

- Left bundle branch block pattern
- Inferior axis (normal or right)
- QRS duration: 0.13 to 0.16 sec
- Responds to adenosine and verapamil

---

[1]A hamartoma is a benign tumorlike nodule that occurs because of an acceleration of growth in a circumscribed area. The nodule is composed of mature cells normally present in the surrounding tissue.

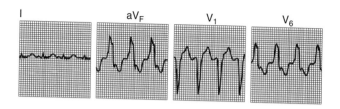

Idiopathic VT with the focus in the right ventricular outflow tract.

Mechanism

May be a heterogenous group with triggered activity as the predominant mechanism; may arise from discrete sites in the free wall of the pulmonary infundibulum.

Idiopathic Left Ventricular Tachycardia
ECG Recognition

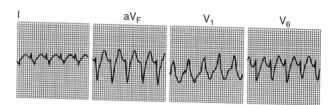

QRS duration: 0.13 to 0.16 sec.
QRS morphology: RBBB pattern.
Axis: Superior, usually left; right in a minority of cases.
Responses: Responds to verapamil; inducibile from the atrium.

Mechanism

Reentry; the origin is in different areas of the left ventricular septum from the base to the midapical region.

Pathology

A false tendon extending from the posteroinferior left ventricle to the septum is a consistent finding.

Bundle Branch Reentrant VT

Sustained bundle branch reentrant VT (BBR-VT) is a highly malignant form of monomorphic VT that frequently presents with syncope, palpitations, or sudden cardiac death.

ECG Recognition

Underlying rhythm: Sinus or atrial fibrillation.
PR interval: Prolonged (in sinus rhythm).
QRS morphology:
- During sinus rhythm: LBBB (incomplete)
- During the VT: Looks like SVT with aberration

Mechanism

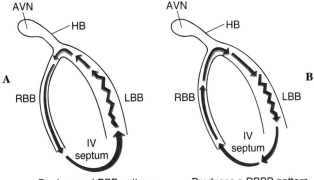

Produces a LBBB pattern   Produces a RBBB pattern

The mechanism of bundle branch reentry VT is schematically depicted. **A,** Its most common form, with anterograde conduction in the RBB to produce an LBBB pattern. The required delay of conduction is evident in the ascending limb of the circuit. **B,** The least common form, with anterograde conduction in the LBBB to produce an RBBB pattern.

The macroreentry circuits of the two forms of bundle branch reentry. Note the slow conduction within the LBBB, a prerequisite for the reentry loop. Other components are the His bundle, RBB, and transseptal ventricular muscle.

Pathophysiology

- Significant structural heart disease, with dilated cardiomyopathy (usually idiopathic) and slow conduction in the His-Purkinje system.
- Dilated ischemic cardiomyopathy
- Nonspecific intraventricular conduction abnormalities
- Dilated ventricles secondary to coronary or significant valvular heart disease
- His-Purkinje system disease

Emergency Treatment

- Unstable patient: DC cardioversion
- Stable patient: Procainamide hydrochloride or lidocaine

Long-Term Treatment

Radiofrequency ablation is a cure, but congestive heart failure is a common cause of death.

Prognosis

Poor; may be considered for cardiac transplantation

Ventricular Flutter and Ventricular Fibrillation

Ventricular flutter and ventricular fibrillation, severe derangements of the electrical rhythm of the heart, are associated with hemodynamic collapse and usually result in death within 3 to 5 minutes without prompt intervention.

ECG Recognition

V$_1$

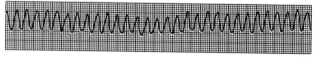

Ventricular flutter. The rate of almost 300 beats/min and the sine wave configuration can be seen.

- Ventricular flutter
QRS/T: Regular large zigzag oscillating pattern
Rate: Ranges from 150 to 300/min

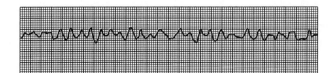

- Ventricular fibrillation

Irregular undulations without clear-cut ventricular complexes

Mechanisms

- Coronary artery disease (most common setting).
- Other clinical settings are hypertension, hyperlipidemia, cigarette smoking, obesity, impaired glucose tolerance, left ventricular hypertrophy, during antiarrhythmic drug administration, hypoxia, ischemia, atrial fibrillation in patients with accessory pathways, and after cardioversion.

Physical Signs

- Often no warning
- Faintness and loss of consciousness
- Blood pressure and pulse cannot be obtained
- Heart sounds: usually absent
- Cyanosis

Treatment

Provide immediate electrical shock.
- DC defibrillation (200–400 joules); the earlier the better (fewer joules are required if done early).
- After conversion, monitor continuously.

Aberration
Versus Ectopy

14

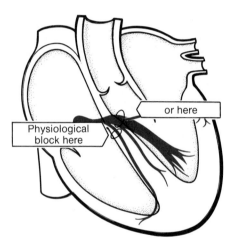

Aberrant ventricular conduction is functional or physiological right or left bundle branch block (RBBB or LBBB) usually caused by shortening of the cycle length.

Misdiagnosis

Misdiagnosis of VT may result in immediate hemodynamic collapse in the acute stage of therapy. If the patient survives and is still misdiagnosed, subsequent mismanagement may result in death. Here's why errors are made:

1. Erroneous perception that SVT with aberrancy is as common as VT

2. In hemodynamic stability, a clinician's wrong assumption that VT is unlikely
3. Failure to thoroughly analyze the 12-lead ECG, take a history, and do a physical examination
4. Ignorance of the morphological clues that identify ventricular tachycardia (VT)
5. Inability to differentiate T waves from P waves in the broad QRS tachycardia

ECG in Aberrancy

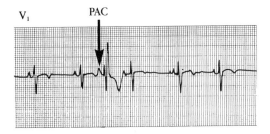

- PAC with RBBB aberrancy; note the rSR pattern and initiating PAC.

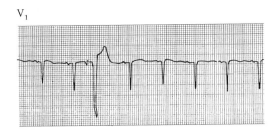

- PAC with LBBB aberrancy; note the relatively narrow QS pattern and initiating PAC.

ECG in Ventricular Ectopy

ECG Signs of AV Dissociation

II

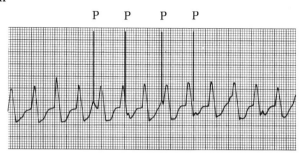

- Ventricular tachycardia with AV dissociation

Independent P waves can be seen throughout the tracing; four of them are marked. Note that these P waves are found because they distort the ECG cycle differently each time.

ECG Signs of VA Conduction

- Ventricular tachycardia with 2:1 retrograde conduction to the atria

Some form of retrograde conduction to the atria occurs 50% of the time during VT (the P′ waves are negative in the leads II, III, and aVF; and positive in lead aVR).

V_1

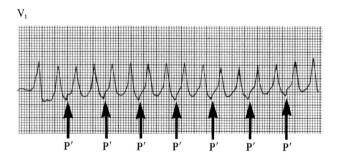

- Ventricular tachycardia with 2:1 retrograde conduction. Note the negative P′ waves in every other T wave.

Leads of Choice

All 12 leads are best; 5 leads are second best (V_1, V_2, and V_6 for morphological clues and leads I and II or aV_F for axis).

QRS Width

A QRS of more than 0.14 seconds is highly suggestive of VT.

QRS Morphology When V_1 is Positive

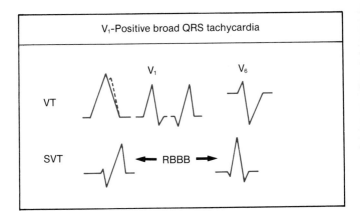

Morphological signs of SVT:
1. Triphasic pattern of RBBB (rSR′ in V_1 and qRs in V_6)
2. QRS of less than 0.14 secs
3. R:S ratio in V_6 greater than 1 (R > S)

Morphological signs of VT:
1. Monophasic or diphasic complex (R, qR, or RS) in lead V_1
2. The "rabbit ear" sign in V_1 (Rr′)
3. An R:S ratio in V_6 greater than 1

QRS Morphology When V_1 is Negative

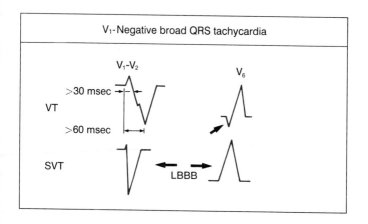

Morphological signs of SVT:

1. Small, narrow r wave in V_1, V_2, or both during LBBB aberration, if an r wave is present
2. Swift smooth S downstroke in V_1 and V_2, reflecting conduction in the His-Purkinje system
3. Early S nadir in V_1 and V_2, less than or equal to 0.06 sec from the onset of the QRS

Morphological signs of VT:

1. Wide R in V_1, V_2, or both (>0.03 sec)
2. Slurred S downstroke (V_1, V_2, or both)
3. Delayed S nadir (V_1, V_2, or both) (>0.06 sec)
4. Any Q in V_6; confirms VT, but *only* if the complex is mainly negative in V_1. This clue cannot be applied to the tachycardia that is positive in V_1.

Warning: QRS morphology can be misleading if the entire clinical setting is not considered. SVT is morphologically identical to VT when there is an accessory pathway and with drugs that slow intraventricular conduction. VT types that can be mistaken for SVT with aberration are fascicular VT, idiopathic VT, and BB reentrant VT.

Is Axis Determination Useful?

Axis diagnostic of VT:

- "No man's land" ($-90°$ to $\pm180°$); sometimes also called northwest quadrant or "indeterminate"
- Right axis when V_1 is negative

Supportive of VT:

- Abnormal axis when V_1 is positive

Not helpful:

- Left axis deviation when V_1 is negative

Clinical Correlations of Axis:

Previous myocardial infarction: Usually abnormal and often superior (negative complex in aV_F). This is especially true when V_1 is positive.

Idiopathic VT: Usually marked left or right axis, but may be normal.

Preexisting BBB: A markedly abnormal axis may occur in SVT.

Right or posteroseptal accessory pathway: Marked left axis in SVT.

Left lateral accessory pathway: Marked right axis in SVT.

Class IC drugs: Marked left axis.

Value of a Baseline 12-Lead ECG

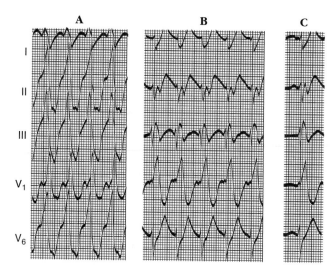

Electrocardiograms from a 15-year-old boy who had complete correction of Fallot's tetralogy. **A** and **B,** A tachycardia with a wide QRS complex; **C,** sinus rhythm with RBBB and left axis deviation. During programmed stimulation the tachycardia in **A** was found to be ventricular and the one in **B** originated in the AV node (SVT). The shape of the QRS, **B,** is identical to the shape of the sinus rhythm, **C.** These ECGs demonstrate that if a patient is admitted in tachycardia showing the recording of **B,** the clinician probably would make the incorrect diagnosis of VT. They demonstrate the necessity of careful comparison with the ECG during sinus rhythm in patients with wide QRS during tachycardia.

(C, from Wellens HJJ et al. In Josephson ME, ed: Ventricular tachycardia: mechanisms and management, Mount Kisco, NY, 1982, Futura.)

In VT and preexisting BBB (right or left), the QRS morphology during the tachycardia is clearly different from that recorded during sinus rhythm, whereas in SVT the morphology is usually identical to that of the sinus rhythm.

Capture Beats and Fusion Beats

Capture, in the context of the broad QRS tachycardia, refers to the unexpected conduction of a sinus beat to the ventricles during VT. *Fusion* refers to the simultaneous activation of the ventricles (or atria) by two foci. A fusion beat or a capture beat is strong evidence of VT, but it is not diagnostic. Fusion beats and capture beats are also seen in the broad QRS tachycardia of supraventricular origin (atrial fibrillation with conduction over an accessory pathway or sinus tachycardia with BBB and end-diastolic VPBs).

Concordant Pattern

Negative precordial concordance is usually diagnostic of VT; positive precordial concordance is supportive.

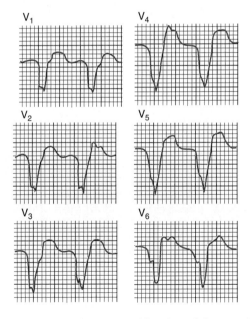

Negative precordial concordance. The slurred downstroke in lead V_1 and the delayed S nadir in leads V_1 and V_2 (discussed on p. 132) are also evident.

Negative precordial concordance reflects a focus in the anteroapical left ventricle.

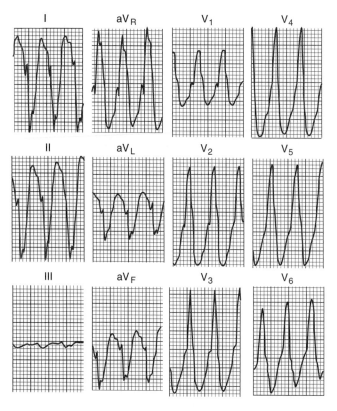

Positive precordial concordance caused by VT. The axis from −90 to ±180 degrees ("no man's land") can also be seen.

Positive precordial concordance results when ventricular activation originates in the posterobasal left ventricle or from SVT with an accessory pathway located in that region. However, because positive precordial concordance caused by SVT is rare, the finding should raise the level of suspicion for VT.

Steps in the Differential Diagnosis

- Take a history.
  Prior MI? *Yes* signals VT.
  "Palpitations" started only after the infarction? *Yes* indicates VT.
- Look for the physical and ECG signs of AV dissociation.
- Look for the ECG signs of ventriculoatrial (VA) conduction.
- Evaluate the QRS configuration, width, and axis.
- Look for precordial concordance, capture beats, and fusion beats.
- When in doubt, use procainamide hydrochloride; if rate does not slow and rhythm convert, cardiovert and refer for evaluation.

Actions of Procainamide Hydrochloride

- Slows the rate of the VT, partially compensating for the fall in blood pressure
- Antifibrillatory
- Drug of choice for nonischemic VT
- Slows conduction in accessory pathways
- Slows conduction in the retrograde direction in fast AV nodal pathway (terminates PSVT)

Physical Signs of AV Dissociation

- Irregular cannon 'a' waves in the jugular pulse
- Varying intensity of the first heart sound
- Beat-to-beat changes in systolic blood pressure
  Any one of these clues indicates AV dissociation, although their absence does not rule out either VT or AV dissociation itself (e.g., VT with atrial fibrillation would have none of these signs).

Summary

When differentiating between aberrant ventricular conduction and ventricular ectopy, keep in mind the following:
1. VT is more common than SVT with aberration.
2. VT is frequently associated with structural heart disease and previous MI.
3. When in doubt, do not use verapamil; use procainamide hydrochloride.
4. A correct diagnosis can generally be made from the surface ECG when all criteria are applied.

Highly reliable ECG criteria for VT:

- AV dissociation
- Fusion beats
- Capture beats
- QRS duration greater than 0.14 sec in V_1-positive patterns
- QRS duration greater than 0.16 sec in V_1-negative patterns
- Precordial QRS concordance (negative is diagnostic; positive is very supportive)
- Axis of −90 degrees to ±180 degrees
- Right axis deviation in V_1-negative broad QRS tachycardia
- QRS morphology in tachycardia unlike that in sinus rhythm with BBB
- In V_1-negative patterns, a broad R, slurred S downstroke, and delayed S nadir in V_1, V_2, or both; or a Q wave in V_6
- In V_1-positive patterns, a monophasic R or biphasic complex (qR; RS), or taller left "rabbit ear" in V_1

Highly reliable ECG criteria for SVT:

- QRS duration of 0.14 sec or less in V_1-positive patterns
- QRS duration of 0.16 sec or less in V_1-negative patterns
- QRS morphology in tachycardia same as that in sinus rhythm with BBB
- In V_1-negative patterns, a narrow r and clean S downstroke in V_1 and V_2
- In V_1-positive patterns, a triphasic pattern in V_1

Polymorphic Ventricular Tachycardia

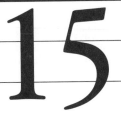

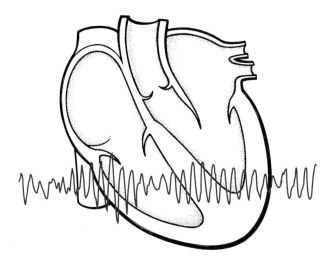

Polymorphic ventricular tachycardia has a continuously changing QRS complex morphology and a more ominous prognosis than that of sustained monomorphic VT. Recognition of this life-threatening arrhythmia is important because it is not treated like other VTs. It can be exacerbated by the administration of class IA drugs, some class IC drugs, and sotalol hydrochloride, but it responds to intravenous magnesium and possibly class IB drugs.

Classification

Polymorphic VT is classified according to whether the QT (or QTU) interval is normal or prolonged. The term *torsades de pointes* (TdP) is reserved exclusively for the type of polymorphic VT associated with a prolonged QT interval.

The Corrected QT (QTc) Interval

The QT interval lengthens with bradycardia and shortens with tachycardia, so it may be corrected for heart rate (QTc), using a 1920 formula introduced by Bazett (QTc = QT/square root of the RR interval). Some computer readouts give the QTc, in which case it is necessary only to know the normal QT (0.39 ± 0.4 sec) to evaluate QT prolongation.

Polymorphic VT with Prolonged QT

 ## Torsades de Pointes

TdP is a rapid polymorphic VT with a distinctive, twisting configuration, associated with prolonged repolarization. It may be acquired (iatrogenic) or congenital.

ECG Recognition

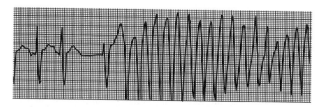

Torsades de pointes (continuous strip). The long QT interval with the U wave distorting it, the pause before the onset of the tachycardia, and the typical undulating, spindle appearance of the pattern are evident.
From the late Dr. Alan Lindsay collection, Salt Lake City, Utah.

• Initiation is pause-dependent (short-long-short preceding cycles).
• Pattern undulates.

- Heart rate is 200 to 250 beats/min.
- QT prolongation exists and is usually more than 0.50 sec in the sinus beats preceding the tachycardia.

Causes

- Potassium channel blockers
- Bradycardia
- Hypokalemia
- Erythromycin
- Antihistamines

Mechanism

The concatenation of events leading to acquired TdP are (1) hypokalemia, (2) prolongation of the action potential duration, (3) early afterdepolarizations, and (4) the critically slow conduction that contributes to reentry. The early afterdepolarizations initiate the tachycardia; the reentry sustains it.

Emergency Treatment

1. Provide continuous monitoring.
2. Discontinue all potentially responsible agents.
3. Give IV potassium.
4. Give IV magnesium, if unsuccessful; then:
5. Overdrive ventricular pacing or isoproterenol may increase the basic heart rate and thus shorten the QT interval. (Isoproterenol is contraindicated in patients with hypertension or ischemic heart disease.)
6. Temporary ventricular or atrial pacing suppresses the VT, and it may remain abated after pacing is discontinued.
7. Direct current cardioversion is usually transiently effective.

Possible Outcomes

- Slowing and then spontaneous conversion
- Conversion and then a new attack
- Ventricular standstill
- Ventricular fibrillation

Contraindications for Magnesium

- Renal failure
- Disappearance of deep tendon reflex
- Rise in serum Mg above 5 mEq/L
- Drop in systolic blood pressure below 80 mg
- Drop in pulse below 60 beats/min

Prevention

After initiation of drugs that prolong the QT interval, take the following steps:

1. Monitor the QT interval.
2. Modify the dosage of the drug if the QT interval reaches 0.56 to 0.60 sec.
3. Discontinue the drug, and hospitalize the patient immediately if the patient complains of lightheadedness or syncope or if you note increased frequency and complexity of PVCs.
4. Screen for congenital TdP.

⩗ Congenital Long QT Syndrome

Congenital (chromosome 7–linked) long QT syndrome (LQTS) results from mutations in a recently cloned gene (HERG) that encodes subunits that form one of the human potassium channels (I_{Kr}).

ECG Recognition

- Prolongation of the QT interval
- Abnormal T wave morphology
- Biphasic, bifid, or notched T waves, particularly in the precordial leads
- Increased QT interval dispersion on the 12-lead ECG
- Abnormal ST-T wave morphology
- T wave alternans
- Abnormal QT/RR interval slope
- Abnormal QRST isoarea distribution

Physical Signs

- Syncope
- Sudden death

Emergency Treatment

- β-blockade.
- Permanent pacing.
- Left cardiac sympathetic denervation.

  (None of the above correct the repolarization abnormality.)

- Potassium has been found to be effective in shortening the QT interval.

Polymorphic VT without Prolonged QT

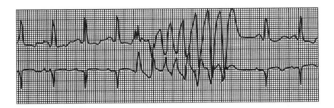

- From a patient with stable coronary artery disease and prior myocardial damage, but no evidence of acute ischemia

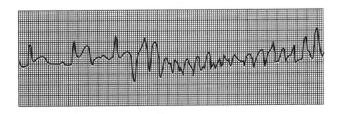

- From a patient with acute myocardial ischemia

Accelerated Idioventricular Rhythm and Ventricular Escape

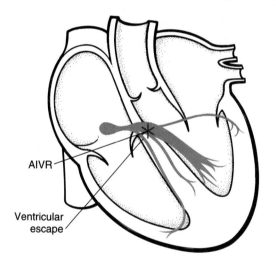

AIVR

Ventricular escape

Accelerated Idioventricular Rhythm

An *accelerated idioventricular rhythm* (AIVR) consists of three or more successive ventricular beats with a rate between 50 and 120 beats/min. It begins with a long coupling interval.

ECG Recognition of AIVR During Reperfusion

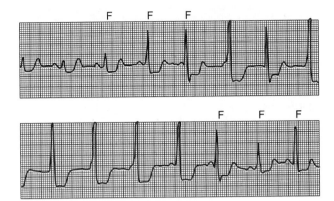

Accelerated idioventricular rhythm (AIVR). Note the fusion (F) beats at the onset of the tachycardia and at the end of this continuous tracing. The rate of the tachycardia is approximately that of the sinus rhythm, which explains the fusion beats at the onset and at the end.

Because its rate is so similar to that of the sinus node, there are fusion beats at its beginning and end or even throughout its duration as the two pacemakers (sinus and ventricular) compete for dominance. The AIVR is a sign of reperfusion during acute myocardial infarction.

Rhythm: Transient and intermittent; lasting for three or more successive beats to one minute; may be regular or irregular.

Rate: Faster than the intrinsic escape rate of the ventricles (30–40 beats/min) but slower than VT.

Onset: Gradual (nonparoxysmal) and beginning with a long coupling interval, often with a ventricular fusion beat.

Termination: Gradual, often ending in ventricular fusion beats.

AV dissociation: Common and often isorhythmic.

ECG Identification of the Area of Reperfusion

Left anterior descending coronary artery reperfusion: Multiple QRS configurations during the AIVR and a relatively narrow QRS.

Circumflex reperfusion: Ruled out when V_1 is negative.

Right coronary artery reperfusion: Ruled out when the electrical axis is inferior, between 0 and ± 180 degrees.

ECG Recognition of AIVR *Not* Related to Reperfusion

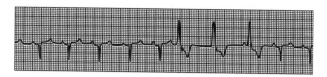

First 24 hours of infarction (after reperfusion): Begins with a short coupling interval but not with fusion beats, although it may end with them.

Possible Mechanisms

- Abnormal automaticity
- Triggered activity
- Related to duration of ischemia (>40 min = AIVR; shorter and reentry type is VT)

Clinical Implications

- Usually benign (even when multiform)
- Of short duration (seconds to a minute)
- Well-tolerated hemodynamically
- Does not seriously affect the clinical course or prognosis
- Associated with acute MI (moment of reperfusion), digitalis toxicity, cocaine intoxication
- Seen in normal hearts
- Reperfusion (50% of patients post-MI; spontaneous or after thrombolytic therapy) and myocardial necrosis

Treatment

Reperfusion arrhythmia: AIVR requires no treatment other than the care of the underlying problem.[1] Reperfusion arrhythmias have not been associated with an increased incidence of ventricular fibrillation or in-hospital mortality.[2]

---

[1]Grimm W, Marchlinski FE: Accelerated idioventricular rhythm, bidirectional ventricular tachycardia. In Zipes DP, Jalife J, editors: *Cardiac electrophysiology from cell to bedside,* Philadelphia, 1995, WB Saunders, pp. 920–926.

[2]Opie LH: Reperfusion injury and its pharmacologic modification, *Circulation* 80:1049, 1989.

Digitalis toxicity: When digitalis is the cause, the drug should be discontinued.

Hemodynamic symptoms: When associated with hemodynamic impairment, the sinus rate may be increased with atropine or atrial pacing. This is usually sufficient to suppress the AIVR. Such hemodynamic symptoms are caused either by the AV dissociation (loss of "atrial kick") or the ventricular rate being too fast.[1,3]

Other conditions: Therapy same as for VT is considered for double tachycardia (AIVR and a more rapid VT) and when AIVR begins with an R-on-T.

Ventricular Escape

Ventricular escape is a beat or rhythm that arises below the branching portion of the His bundle when the junctional escape mechanism fails.

ECG Recognition

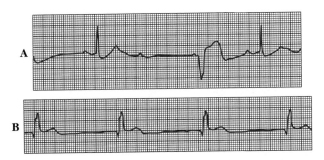

A, Ventricular escape (the second ventricular complex).
B, Slow idioventricular rhythm.

Rate: Less than 40 beats/min.
QRS complex: Broad.
AV block or atrial standstill is present

---

[3]Zipes DP: Specific arrhythmias: diagnosis and treatment. In Braunwald E, editor: *Heart disease,* 4th edition, Philadelphia, 1992, WB Saunders, pp. 667–718.

Digitalis Dysrhythmias

17

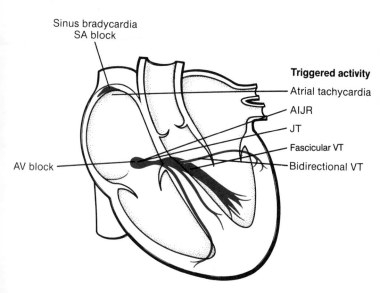

Sinus bradycardia
SA block

Triggered activity
Atrial tachycardia
AIJR
JT
Fascicular VT
Bidirectional VT

AV block

ᴸᴬ Digitalis Glycosides

Digitalis: Derived from the dried leaf of the foxglove plant, *Digitalis purpura.*

Digoxin: Derived from the *Digitalis lanata* plant; digitalis compound most widely used clinically.

Digitoxin: Derived from both of the abovementioned plants; metabolized by an enterohepatic route; serum half-life of 5 to 6 days.

Advantages of Digoxin

- Digoxin persistently increases the ejection fraction during long-term administration in patients with heart failure.
- Therapeutic benefit is on par with diuretics and ACE inhibitors in symptomatic heart failure.
- Digoxin increases vagal activity, slowing conduction through the AV node. It is useful in controlling the ventricular response to atrial tachyarrhythmias.
- Digoxin is inexpensive.
- It is hemodynamically tolerated.
- It is easy to administer.

Disadvantages of Digoxin

- Narrow therapeutic window
- Possibility of toxicity preceding the desired therapeutic effect
- Difficulty in acutely titrating the dose to achieve a predictable heart rate in atrial fibrillation
- Significant interactions with other drugs used to treat atrial fibrillation (e.g., verapamil, quinidine, procainamide hydrochloride)
- Inability to control ventricular response in atrial fibrillation, in the face of heightened sympathetic tone
- Mortality near 100% in unrecognized digitalis toxicity

Systematic Approach to the ECG

- Look for P waves in lead II.
- Determine the atrial rate.
- Commit to a diagnosis of the atrial condition.
- If no P waves are seen (atrial fibrillation), proceed as follows:
- Evaluate for AV dissociation (regular or group beating).
- Switch to V_1 to evaluate for QRS morphology.

Clinical Alert to Digitalis Toxicity

Watch for the following:

- Neurologic symptoms (headache, malaise, neuralgic pain, pseudodementia such as disorientation, memory lapses, hallucinations, nightmares, restlessness, insomnia, and listlessness)
- Changes in the quality of color vision, especially red and green (ask patient about change in quality of TV color)
- Gastrointestinal symptoms (mediated by chemoreceptors in the medulla)

- Bradycardia
    Sinus
    SA block
    AV block
- Tachycardia
    Atrial tachycardia with block
    Junctional tachycardia
    Fascicular VT
- Regularity in atrial fibrillation
    Junctional tachycardia
    AV block with junctional escape
- Group beating in atrial fibrillation
    Junctional tachycardia with Wenckebach exit block
- Group beating in sinus rhythm
    Ventricular bigeminy
    SA Wenckebach
    AV Wenckebach
- Atrial flutter with the following:
    AV dissociation
    High-degree AV block (bradycardia)

Sinus Bradycardia and Junctional Tachycardia

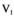

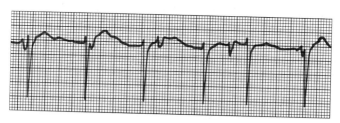

Two of the effects of digitalis toxicity are sinus bradycardia and junctional tachycardia (70 beats/min). Strictly speaking, this is an accelerated idiojunctional rhythm (AIJR).

SA and AV Block
ECG Recognition (SA Wenckebach)

V₂

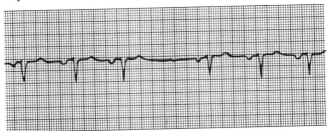

- Group beating (dropped P waves)
- Shortening PP intervals
- Pauses less than twice the shortest PP cycle

ECG Recognition (AV Wenckebach)

II

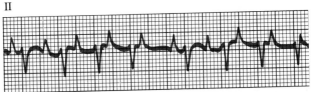

- Group beating
- Lengthening PR intervals
- Shortening RR intervals
- Pauses less than twice the shortest cycle

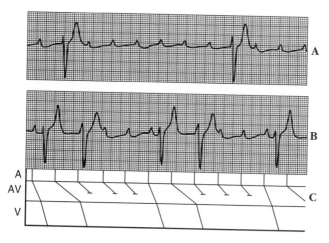

Profound life-threatening bradycardia caused by high-grade AV block in an acute digitalis overdose (suicide attempt). The top tracing was recorded at admission. The middle tracing shows conduction improvement with treatment. The bottom is the laddergram. The broad initial R wave of that beat is really a distortion by a P wave.

Atrial Tachycardia

ECG Recognition

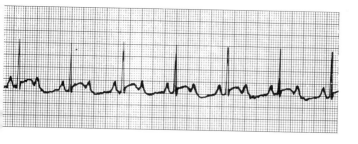

Atrial rate: Dose-related in the range of 130 to 250 beats/min.

AV conduction: Usually 2:1, but sometimes Wenckebach periods. When digitalis is discontinued, conduction improves before the tachycardia converts to sinus rhythm. Thus, there is usually a transient period of 1:1 conduction.

Rhythm: Ventriculophasic behavior of P′P′ intervals (60% of cases); that is, the P′P′ interval containing the R wave is shorter than the P′P′ interval without an R wave.

P′ wave shape: Almost identical to the sinus P waves. The atrial focus is high in the right atrium, near the sinus node, causing the P′ waves to resemble those of sinus rhythm.

Best lead: II (P′ wave easily differentiated from P′ with low atrial foci).

Mortality: 100%.

Junctional Tachycardia

Digitalis overdose has long been considered the most common cause of junctional tachycardia. Other causes are acute myocardial infarction, cardiac surgery, rheumatic fever, chronic obstructive pulmonary disease, and hypokalemia.

ECG Recognition

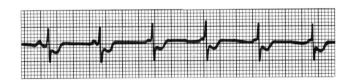

Junctional rate: 70 to 140 beats/min; increases with exercise but rarely exceeds 140 beats/min.

Carotid sinus massage: No effect, or there may be nodoventricular block.

Retrograde conduction: Usually absent because of the AV block created by the digitalis; therefore, AV dissociation is usually present.

Rhythm: Nonparoxysmal accelerated junctional rhythm (gradual onset). The underlying rhythm may be sinus, atrial fibrillation, atrial flutter, or atrial tachycardia (itself a result of digitalis toxicity).

Best lead: V_1; in this lead junctional tachycardia (rS pattern) it can be differentiated from fascicular VT (rSR′ pattern).

Mortality: 80%.

Rhythm Variations

II

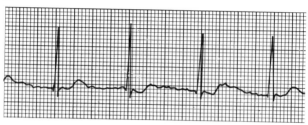

Atrial fibrillation with junctional tachycardia (accelerated idiojunctional rhythm)

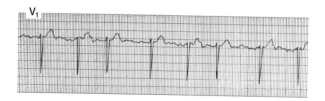

Atrial fibrillation with junctional tachycardia and Wenckebach exit block (group beating)

V_1

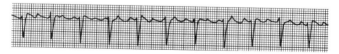

Atrial flutter with junctional tachycardia; note the changing flutter-R relationship (a sign of AV dissociation in atrial flutter when the ventricular rhythm is regular)

Fascicular Ventricular Tachycardia

The focus is in one of the fascicles of the left bundle branch, producing a pattern that resembles incomplete RBBB with axis deviation.

ECG Recognition

V₁

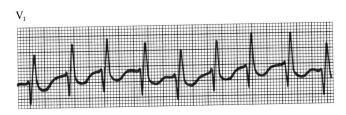

QRS width: Narrower than usual (usually about 0.12 sec).
QRS pattern: RBBB pattern (rSR′ in V_1).
QRS axis: Left (anterior fascicle) or right (posterior fascicle).
Rate: 90 to 160 beats/min.
Mortality: 100%.

Bifascicular Ventricular Tachycardia

This is a life-threatening form of ventricular tachycardia and a manifestation of severe digitalis intoxication. The two fascicles of the left bundle branch alternate pacing the ventricles, resulting in a unique ECG pattern.

ECG Recognition

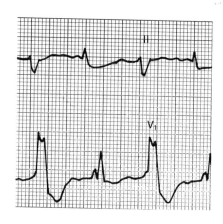

QRS width: Narrower than usual (usually about 0.12 sec).
QRS pattern: RBBB pattern (not the pathology) (rSR' in V_1). There is QRS alternans in V_1 caused by the alternating axes (right and left).
QRS axis: Alternating right and left.
Rate: Usually 90 to 160 beats/min.
Mortality: 100%.

Treatment of Early Stages of Digitalis Toxicity

It may be sufficient to temporarily withdraw the drug until the patient is stabilized. When the arrhythmias become more obtrusive or the patient manifests symptoms, take the following steps:

- Discontinue the digitalis.
- Require bed rest (avoid sympathetic stimulation).
- Correct electrolyte abnormalities.
- Provide continuous ECG monitoring.
- Do a physical assessment.
- Do not use carotid sinus massage (may result in VF).
- Provide ventricular pacing for symptomatic bradycardia.
- Prescribe phenytoin and place a pacing wire for hemodynamic deterioration.

Indications for Digoxin-Specific Antibody Fab Fragments (Digibind)

- Hemodynamic instability
- Hyperkalemia
- AV block
- Malignant ventricular tachyarrhythmias

Atrioventricular Block

18

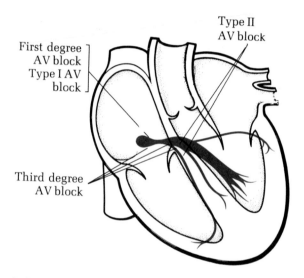

Type II
AV block

First degree
AV block
Type I AV
block

Third degree
AV block

Atrioventricular (AV) block is the delayed conduction or nonconduction of an atrial impulse during a time when the AV junction is not physiologically refractory.

First degree AV block: Prolonged PR intervals.

Second degree AV block: Not all P waves are conducted; divided into type I (AV Wenckebach or Mobitz I), type II (Mobitz II), and 2:1.

High-grade AV block: Block of two or more consecutive P waves.

Third-degree AV block: Absence of AV conduction when the possibility to conduct is present.

First Degree AV Block (Prolonged PR Interval)
ECG Recognition

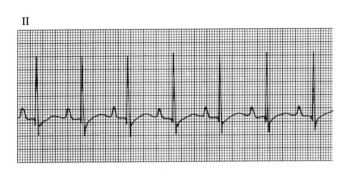

II

PR interval: Longer than 0.20 sec.; does not change from beat to beat.

QRS complex: Normal in shape and duration unless there is another lesion lower in the conduction system. A narrow QRS usually indicates conduction delay within the AV node (prolonged AH interval).

AV conduction: All sinus beats are conducted to the ventricles.

Pathology

- Prolonged PR plus normal QRS: Conduction delay in the AV node
- Prolonged PR plus BBB pattern: AV nodal and/or His-Purkinje pathology
- Occasionally conduction delay within the atria

Clinical Implications

Usually transient in the setting of acute inferior MI.

Pediatrics

In children taking digitalis, the PR may become prolonged, and, unlike in adults, such a development may represent digitalis toxicity.

Bedside Diagnosis

- Long a-c wave interval in the jugular venous pulse.
- Diminished intensity of the first heart sound.

- PR shortens with atropine, exercise, or catecholamines if pathology is AV nodal.
- PR shortens with carotid sinus massage if subnodal.

Treatment

None.

▲⣤ Second Degree AV Block

In second degree AV block, not all atrial impulses are conducted to the ventricles. This may be classified into three categories:

Type I (AV Wenckebach or Mobitz I)
Type II (Mobitz II)
2:1 AV block

Type I (AV Wenckebach)

In classic AV Wenckebach, the PR lengthens until finally one P wave is not conducted, producing a pause. Following the pause, the sequence repeats itself.

ECG Recognition

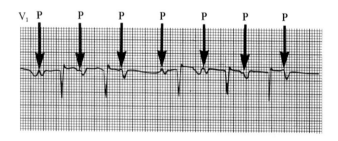

P waves: Sinus.

PR intervals: Lengthen progressively before the dropped beat.

QRS complexes: Narrow unless there is another lesion in the bundle branches.

Rhythm: Group beating (because of the dropped beats).

RR intervals: Shorten if there are more than two P waves in a row conducted.

AV conduction: Improves with atropine, exercise, or catecholamines; worsens with carotid sinus massage when the conduction problem is AV nodal.

Distinguishing features: The footprints of AV Wenckebach are group beating, lengthening PR intervals, shortening RR intervals (when three or more Ps are consecutively conducted), and pauses that are less than twice the shortest cycle.

Rhythm Variations

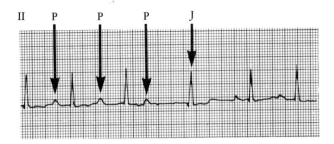

AV Wenckebach with junctional (J) escape

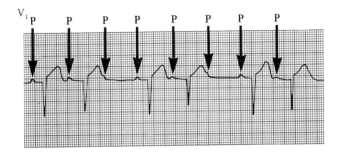

3:2 AV Wenckebach

Pathology

Almost always in the AV node, rarely within the His bundle.

▶ Clinical Implications

Associated with:

- Digitalis toxicity
- Acute inferior MI (identifies high risk)
- Right ventricular MI
- Acute myocarditis
- Post-open heart surgery
- Normal in trained athletes

Bedside Diagnosis

- A widening a-c interval in the jugular venous pulse terminated by a pause
- An *a* wave not followed by a *v* wave
- Gradually diminishing intensity of the first heart sound
- Improved conduction with atropine exercise, or catecholamines

Treatment

None; trained athletes should decondition if symptomatic.

Differential Diagnosis

Concealed junctional extrasystoles can mimic second-degree AV block.

Type II

Dropped P waves against a background of fixed PR intervals.

ECG Recognition

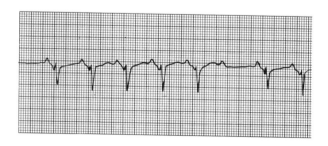

P waves: Sinus; some are not conducted.
PR intervals: The same from beat to beat and usually normal.
QRS complexes: Broad (0.12 sec or more).

Distinguishing features: Recognized because of fixed, normal PR intervals; broad QRS complexes; and dropped beats.

Pathology

The lesion is in the bundle of His or involves both bundle branches. The complete block of one bundle causes the ventricular complexes to be broad; intermittent block of the other bundle causes dropped beats.

Clinical Implications

- Ominous; the physician should be notified.
- Almost always an indication for a pacemaker.
- Often precedes complete AV block and syncope.
- Associated with high-risk anterior septal MI and chronic fibrotic disease of the conduction system.

Bedside Diagnosis

- Intermittent pauses in the heartbeat
- Jugular venous pulse: some *a* waves not followed by *v* waves
- Constant intensity of first heart sound

Treatment

- A temporary pacemaker in the acute setting followed by a permanent pacemaker at a more convenient time.

2 : 1 AV block
ECG Recognition

II

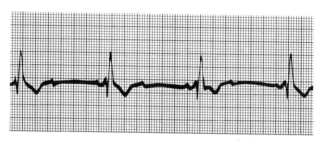

PR intervals: All the same; may be normal (subnodal pathology) or prolonged (AV nodal pathology).
P waves: Sinus.
AV conduction: Two sinus P waves for every QRS.
QRS complex: Narrow (AV nodal pathology) or broad (bundle branch pathology).

Pathology

- AV nodal: Conduction improves with atropine, exercise, or catecholamines and worsens with carotid sinus massage (CSM).
- Subnodal: Conduction improves with CSM and worsens with atropine, exercise, or catecholamines.

Clinical Implications

- Narrow QRS: Associated with acute inferior MI.
- Broad QRS: Associated with acute anterior MI.

Treatment

- Narrow QRS: A pacemaker is usually not necessary.
- Broad QRS: A pacemaker may be indicated in a symptomatic patient.

High-Grade Second Degree AV Block

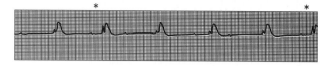

High-grade second degree AV block. There are only two sinus-conducted beats (asterisks), despite a sinus rate of 58 beats/min.

At atrial rates of less than 135 beats/min, two or more consecutive atrial impulses fail to be conducted because of the block itself and not because of interference by an escaping subsidiary pacemaker.

Third Degree (Complete) AV Block

No atrial impulses can be conducted to the ventricles (a form of AV dissociation).

ECG Recognition

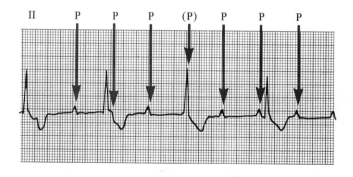

Rate: Less than 40 beats/min in acquired complete block; faster in congenital complete block.

Atrial rhythm: Sinus or ectopic (atrial fibrillation, atrial flutter).

Ventricular rhythm: Independent (may be junctional or ventricular); usually regular, but may be irregular because of PVCs, a pacemaker shift, or autonomic influences.

QRS complex: Depends on the level of block and the condition of the conduction system.

Distinguishing features: Recognized because of AV dissociation and a regular ventricular rhythm of 40 to 60 beats/min.

Rhythm Variations

V_1

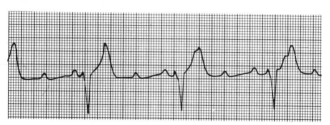

Third degree AV block with an idioventricular rhythm

V_1

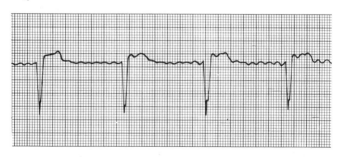

Atrial fibrillation with third degree AV block

Pathology

Complete block at level of AV node (narrow QRS); His bundle (narrow QRS); or bundle branches (broad QRS).

Clinical Implications and Causes

- Chronic degenerative conduction disease
- Digitalis toxicity
- Myocardial infarction

Physical Signs

Presyncope, syncope, or angina.

Treatment

In patients with symptomatic bradyarrhythmias, a temporary or permanent pacemaker is indicated. Appropriate drugs may be used until adequate pacing therapy can be initiated or if the block is likely to be temporary.

Potassium Derangements

19

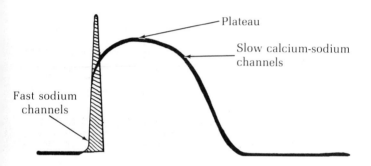

Plateau

Slow calcium-sodium channels

Fast sodium channels

Potassium is excreted by the body in urine, feces, and perspiration. Diuretics, vomiting, diaphoresis, and diarrhea can rapidly deplete the body of this vital ion (hypokalemia). Conversely, anuria can cause a potassium buildup (hyperkalemia). Both conditions may produce serious arrhythmias and even death.

Major Cellular Antiarrhythmic Functions of Potassium

- Determines conduction velocity by helping to create a negative transmembrane potential
- Protects the heart by preventing the QT interval from being too short
- Accommodates rapid heart rates by shortening the QT interval
- Protects excitability in cases of hyperpolarization
- Slows the heart rate in response to vagal stimulation

Hyperkalemia

Mild: Less than 6.5 mEq/L
Moderate: 6.5 to 8 mEq/L
Severe: Greater than 8 mEq/L

ECG Recognition

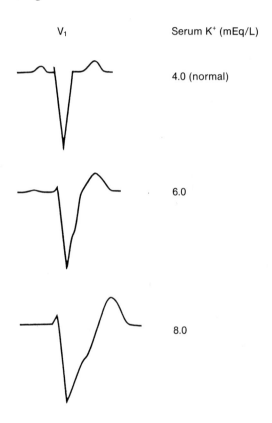

V_1

Serum K^+ (mEq/L)

4.0 (normal)

6.0

8.0

5.7 mEq/L:
- Tall tented T waves.
- T waves often symmetrical with a narrow base.
- Best seen in leads II, III, V_2, and V_4.

6.5 to 8 mEq/L:
- QRS broadens and shows marked slurring of its second portion.
- Wide S wave in left precordial leads.
- QRS axis left.
- ST segment deviates or disappears (terminal S wave becomes continuous with the tall tented T wave).

7 mEq/L:
- P wave amplitude and duration decreases.

Greater than 8 mEq/L:
- P wave duration increases, prolonging the PR interval.
- P wave eventually disappears.
- QRS broadens and becomes continuous with the T wave.
- QRS axis is left.

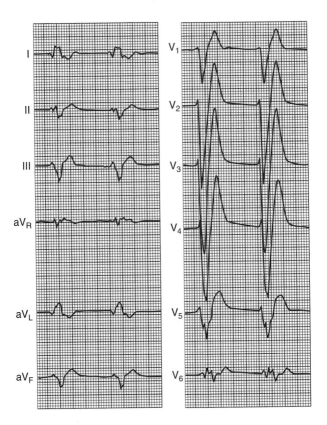

Courtesy Hein JJ Wellers, M.D.

Life-threatening hyperkalemia. Note absence of P waves, broad QRS, left axis shift, lack of ST segment (V₁ to V₅), and peaked T waves.

Treatment

Mild hyperkalemia: Identify and eliminate the cause, if possible (usually renal disease).

Moderate or severe hyperkalemia:

- IV calcium gluconate (10%) 10 to 30 ml IV infusion over 1 to 5 min with constant ECG monitoring. *Effect:* Immediately and briefly alters the effects of the excess potassium on the cellular membranes without lowering the plasma potassium concentration.

- IV glucose solution (10%) 200 to 500 ml in 30 min, and 500 to 1000 ml over the next several hours.
- Sodium bicarbonate (2 to 3 ampules) added to the liter of 5% dextrose in 0.9% saline. *Effect:* IV calcium gluconate and sodium bicarbonate decrease the effect of potassium toxicity by shifting potassium into the cells, even in patients who are not acidotic.
- Cation exchange resins.
- Renal failure: Hemodialysis or peritoneal dialysis.

⩗ Hypokalemia
ECG Recognition

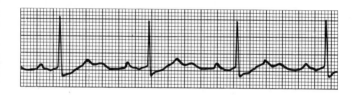

Initially:
   ST segment: Progressive depression.
   T wave: Progressive decrease in amplitude.
Advanced stage:
   QRS interval: Increased amplitude and duration.
   P wave: Increased amplitude and duration.
   PR interval: Slight prolongation.
   Arrhythmias: Bradycardia, AV block, atrial flutter, and an exaggeration of digitalis toxicity.
   Distinguishing features: The U wave gets taller and taller and fuses with the T wave. There is progressive ST depression and decreased T wave amplitude.

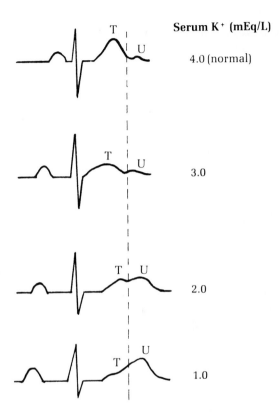

4 mEq/L: Normal U wave is same polarity as T wave and of low amplitude

3 mEq/L: T wave and U wave are same amplitude

2 mEq/L: U wave is taller than T wave

1 mEq/L: Giant U wave fuses with T wave

Causes

- Frank loss of total body potassium through the kidneys or intestines (from use of diuretics, renal disease, adrenal disease, diarrhea).
- Potassium shift from the extracellular to intracellular compartments without a deficit in total body potassium (from infusion of glucose, alkali, large quantities of cortisol or glucocorticoids).
- Both total body loss and cellular shift (vomiting and nasogastric drainage). As hydrochloric acid is lost from the stomach, the body generates bicarbonate, the excess of which is excreted by the kidneys *along with potassium.* The potassium shifts from the extracellular fluid into the cells because of the alkalosis created by the generation of bicarbonate.

Signs and Symptoms

Muscular: Weakness and atrophy.

Neurological: Tetany.

Cerebral: Irritability, lethargy, hallucinations, apathy, drowsiness, confusion, delirium, and coma (the electroencephalogram is usually normal).

Gastrointestinal: Nausea, vomiting, ileus.

Carbohydrate metabolism: Impairment of glucose tolerance.

Renal: Secondary to inability to concentrate urine (nocturia, polyuria, and polydipsia) or inability to maximally acidify urine because of stimulation of the production of massive amounts of renal ammonia by the hypokalemic kidney.

Treatment

- Continuous ECG monitoring
- Repeated measurement of potassium blood levels
- Evaluation for physical signs of hypokalemia (muscular weakness or paralysis)
- Increased dietary intake of potassium salts when possible

For severe potassium deficiency: Give IV potassium chloride (40–60 mEq/L concentrations at 20 mEq/hr, approximately 200–250 mEq/day).

AV Dissociation

20

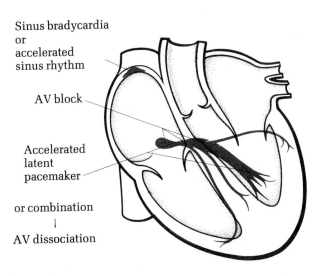

Sinus bradycardia
or
accelerated
sinus rhythm

AV block

Accelerated
latent
pacemaker

or combination
↓
AV dissociation

AV Dissociation

AV dissociation is the independent beating of atria and ventricles. It is never a primary disorder but is always the result of a basic disturbance in impulse formation or conduction.

ECG Recognition

Rate: That of the ventricular pacemaker.

Rhythm: Usually regular, but may be irregular if there is occasional conduction (capture).

QRS duration: Narrow or broad, depending on the ventricular pacemaker.

Distinguishing features: Independently beating atria and ventricles. In some cases, the P waves may appear to "walk into" R waves as the PR interval becomes shorter and shorter.

Rhythm Variations

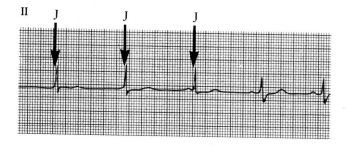

Sinus bradycardia with a junctional escape rhythm

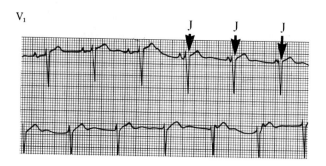

Accelerated idiojunctional rhythm

V₁

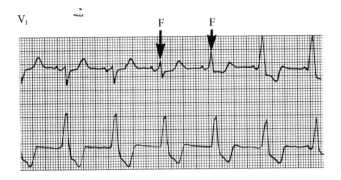

Accelerated idioventricular rhythm (F = fusion beat)

II

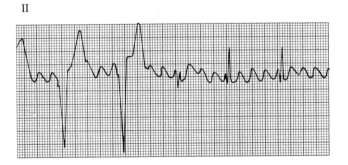

Atrial flutter with an accelerated idioventricular rhythm. (The last three are capture beats, the first of which is a fusion beat.)

II

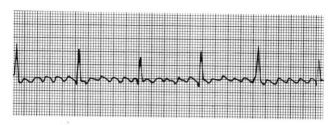

Atrial flutter with AV dissociation and two capture beats (first and fifth)

II

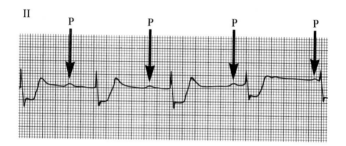

Complete AV block

V₁

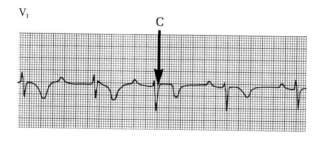

High-grade second-degree AV block with an idiojunctional pacemaker and one capture beat

Causes

- Sinus bradycardia or sinus arrhythmia with a junctional escape rhythm (not abnormal)
- Acceleration of a latent pacemaker: nonparoxysmal junctional tachycardia, accelerated idioventricular rhythm, or ventricular tachycardia (all pathological)
- Complete AV block
- Any combination of these

Physical Findings

- Jugular pulse: Irregular cannon *a* waves
- Heart sounds: Varying intensity of S_1
- Systolic blood pressure: Beat-to-beat changes

Any one indicates AV dissociation, although their absence does not rule it out

Treatment

That of the underlying cause

Fusion Beats

21

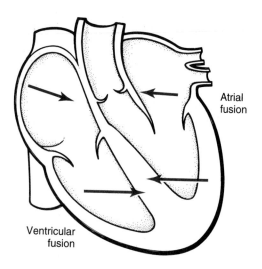

Atrial fusion

Ventricular fusion

A fusion beat is the result of two vectors from two different foci colliding within the muscle mass of either the ventricle (ventricular fusion) or the atria (atrial fusion).

Mechanisms

When two opposing currents collide, they cancel each other out, causing a complex that is narrower or of lower amplitude than the ectopic beat alone.

Ventricular Fusion

ECG Recognition

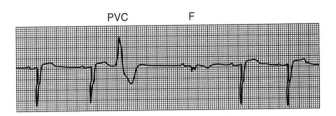

Ventricular fusion (F)
- PVCs are present in tracing.
- QRS complexes are of lower amplitude and/or shorter duration than like ectopic beats.
- May be slightly premature.
- PR interval of the fusion beat may be shorter or the same as that of the underlying sinus rhythm.

Rhythm Variations

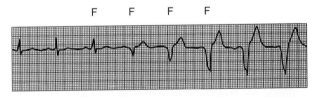

An accelerated idioventricular rhythm. Note the changing shape of the fusion beats (F) as the ventricular ectopic focus dominates more completely with each beat.

Accelerated idioventricular rhythm begins with fusion beats (F).

MCL₁

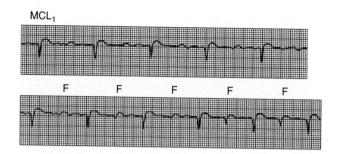

Bigeminal end-diastolic PVCs that are all fusion beats (F)

Atrial Fusion
ECG Recognition

III

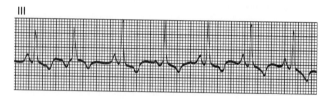

Atrial fusion resulting from atrial parasystole. The fourth P wave is a fusion beat. The laddergram below the tracing depicts the mechanism. The atrial parasystolic focus is circled in the atrial (A) tier; note that the first atrial parasystolic force completely captures the atria, the second is a fusion beat, and the third is not manifested at all because of a preceding sinus beat and atrial refractoriness. In A tier, the sinus-conducted beats slant down and forward. Atrioventricular conduction is depicted in the AV tier. Ventricular conduction is normal, as shown in the V tier.
From the Dr. Alan Lindsay Collection.

- PACs are present in tracing.
- P waves are of lower amplitude and/or shorter duration than like ectopic beats or sinus beats.
- May or may not be slightly premature.
- PR interval of the fusion beat is the same or a little longer than that of the underlying sinus rhythm.

Parasystole

22

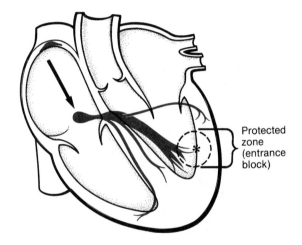

Protected
zone
(entrance
block)

Parasystole is an irregularity caused by a focus of altered automaticity or triggered activity surrounded by an abnormal area of protection, but which may be subject to *electrotonic modulation.*

ECG in Classical Parasystole

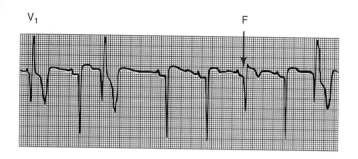

longer intervals. Failure of the parasystolic impulse to appear when expected is called *exit block.*

ECG in Modulated Parasystole

Ventricular ectopics: No fixed coupling; fusion beats.

Interectopic intervals: The regular rhythm of the parasystolic focus is disrupted by subthreshold electrotonic depolarizations transmitted across the depressed barrier, prolonging or shortening the parasystolic cycle.

ECG in Atrial Parasystole

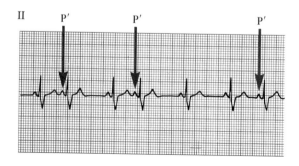

Atrial ectopics: No fixed coupling; fusion beats.

Interectopic intervals: Minimal interval is an exact multiple of longer intervals.

Clinical Implications

- Benign
- Generally not treated

Wolff-Parkinson-White and Other Preexcitation Syndromes

23

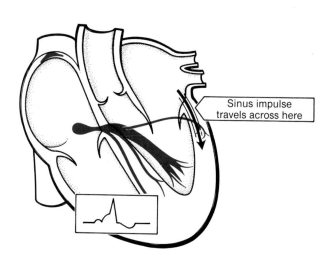

Sinus impulse travels across here

Wolff-Parkinson-White (WPW) syndrome is a group of ECG findings (short PR, delta wave, and broad QRS) associated with the occurrence of tachycardias.

ECG Recognition During Sinus Rhythm

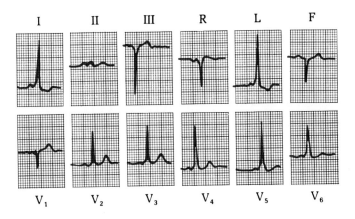

PR interval: Less than 0.12 sec.

QRS complex: Greater than 0.10 sec.

T wave: Secondary changes may be present.

Associated arrhythmias: PSVT and atrial fibrillation.

Ventricular fusion: Nodal-His bundle axis and delta force.

Possible ECG changes:

- Abnormal Q waves
- Slurring of the ascending limb of the R wave
- Increased voltage of the QRS complex
- Axis shift

Anatomical Substrate

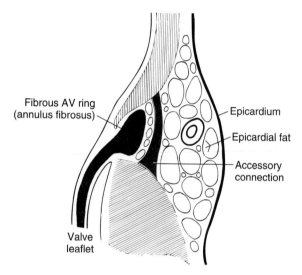

Diagramatic representation of a left-sided accessory atrioventricular (AV) connection. The connection skirts through the epicardial fat, being outside the fibrous AV ring.
From Becker AE et al: *Circulation* 57:870, 1978.

An accessory pathway or AV connection is an extra muscle bundle composed of working myocardial tissue that forms a connection between atria and ventricles outside the conduction system.

Latent Accessory Pathway

There is no preexcitation during sinus rhythm, although the accessory pathway is capable of both anterograde and retrograde conduction.

Concealed Accessory Pathway

There is no preexcitation during sinus rhythm or during supraventricular arrhythmias, since anterograde conduction does not take place in the accessory pathway. Retrograde conduction does, however, occur, and it supports PSVT.

Assessment of the Accessory Pathway Refractory Period

This period is long enough to protect the patient from excessive ventricular rates should atrial fibrillation develop if the following are true:

1. Preexcitation is intermittent.
2. Preexcitation disappears (not just lessens) in all 12 leads with exercise.
3. The PR and QRS normalize following IV procainamide hydrochloride (in a setting where complete heart block can be managed and after ruling out hypertrophic cardiomyopathy).

Two Most Common Arrhythmias in WPW Syndrome

- Orthodromic circus movement tachycardia (Chapter 11)
- Atrial fibrillation

Atrial Fibrillation with Preexcitation

Atrial fibrillation is the second most common arrhythmia in patients with WPW syndrome. It results in a rapid, irregular broad QRS tachycardia that, without intervention, may deteriorate into ventricular fibrillation.

ECG Features

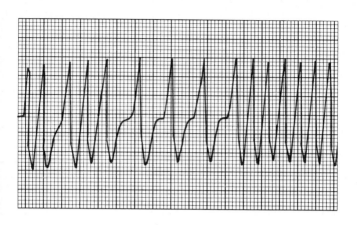

Rate: Fast, usually more than 200 beats/min.
QRS: Broad.
Rhythm: Irregular.
Distinguishing features: A fast, broad, irregular rhythm (FBI), identical to VT, except for its irregularity.

Mechanism

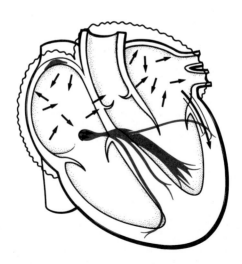

The frequent and erratic atrial impulses of atrial fibrillation are conducted into the ventricles over the accessory pathway. The rapid ventricular rate is determined by the refractory period of the accessory pathway, which varies among individuals. If the refractory period of the accessory pathway is short, the heart rate exceeds 300/min.

Emergency Treatment

- Establish a 12-lead ECG before and after cardioversion.
- If hemodynamically unstable, complete DC cardioversion.
- If hemodynamically stable, provide procainamide hydrochloride at 10 mg/kg body weight over 5 minutes. If the rate does not slow, complete DC cardioversion.
- Refer patient for radiofrequency ablation.
- **Danger:** Do not use digitalis or calcium channel blockers; they may accelerate the ventricular rate.

Symptoms of Arrhythmias

- Palpitations (97%; usually delayed until adolescence or adulthood)
- Dyspnea (57%)
- Anginal pain (56%)
- Perspiration (55%)
- Fatigue (41%)
- Anxiety (30%)
- Dizziness (30%)
- Polyuria (26%)

Nodoventricular and Fasciculoventricular (Mahaim) Fibers

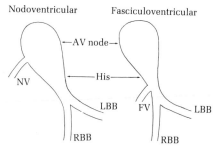

Site of origin:	AV node	His bundle or bundle branches
PR:	Short or normal	Normal (isolated FV)
QRS:	Anomalous—fusion	Anomalous—fixed

From Gallagher JJ et al: Role of Mahaim fibers in cardiac arrhythmias in man, *Circulation* 64:176, 1981. By permission of the American Heart Association, Inc.

Mahaim fibers are congenital anomalous AV connections between the AV node, His bundle, or bundle branches to the ventricles.

ECG During Sinus Rhythm

PR interval: Short or normal (nodoventricular connection); normal (fasciculoventricular connection).

QRS complex: Fusion beat; varies in morphology (nodoventricular connection); anomalous (fasciculoventricular connection).

Mechanism of PSVT (Nodoventricular Fibers)

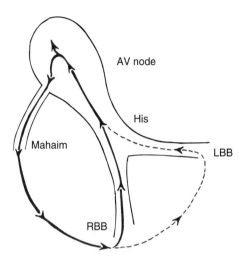

Schematic representation of the reentry circuit underlying a reciprocating tachycardia. This reentry circuit uses a nodoventricular fiber. The nodoventricular fiber may insert into either the right ventricle or the RBB. The retrograde return circuit can conceivably be completed by either the RBB or the LBB. A portion of the reentry loop is confined to the AV node, and the atrium does not form a necessary link in the loop.
From Gallagher JJ et al: *Circulation* 64:176, 1981.

Note that the ventricles are activated outside the conduction system, producing a broad QRS tachycardia.

Short PR Syndrome (Lown-Ganong-Levine Syndrome)

ECG Recognition

- Short PR interval
- Normal QRS duration
- Tendency to AV-reciprocating tachycardia, atrial fibrillation, or atrial flutter

Wellens Syndrome and Left Main and Three-Vessel Disease

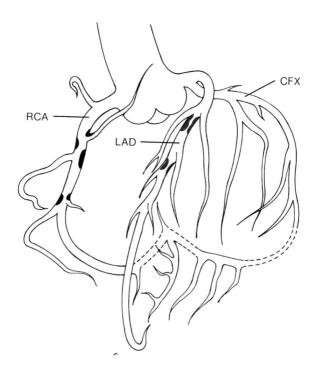

Wellens Syndrome

Wellens syndrome is a group of five signs in a patient with unstable angina that permits ECG recognition of critical proximal LAD stenosis:

- Unstable angina
- Progressive, symmetrical, deep T wave inversion in V_2 and V_3 during pain-free periods
- Little or no enzyme elevation
- Little or no ST segment elevation (≤ 1 mm)
- No loss of precordial R waves

ECG Recognition

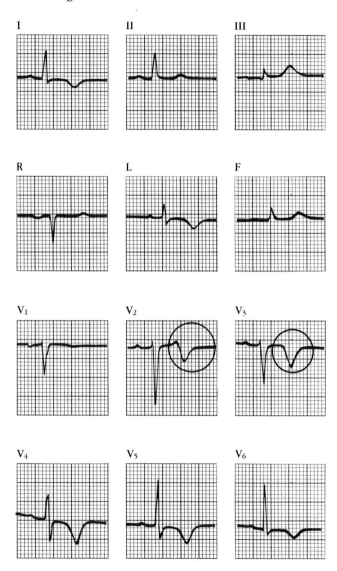

Monitoring Leads

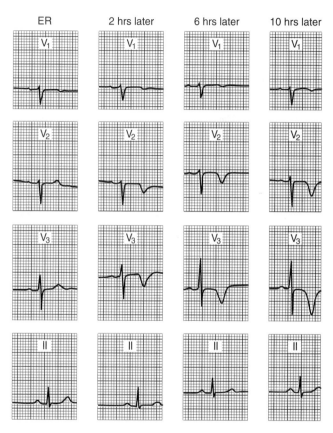

The two diagnostic leads for Wellens syndrome are unquestionably leads V_2 and V_3. Classic picture of progressive, symmetric, deep inversion of the T wave in leads V_2 and V_3 in a patient with 97% occlusion of the proximal LAD. The T waves in leads V_1 and II do not change significantly.

Patients with unstable angina are monitored on lead V_2 or V_3 (MCL$_2$ or MCL$_3$ may be used). Note that in these concurrent serial tracings, the more-traditional monitoring leads (II and V_1) are not diagnostic of this condition.

Mechanism

The T wave inversion of Wellens syndrome represents reperfusion. During chest pain, these T wave changes are replaced by positive T waves with either ST segment elevation or depression. It is during chest pain that the coronary vessel is critically narrowed or occluding.

The ECG During Pain

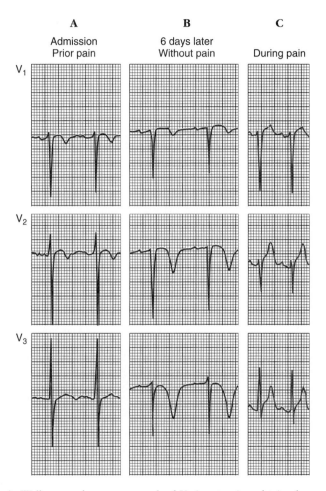

A, Wellens syndrome seen on lead V_2 in a tracing obtained on admission. **B,** During pain, the ST segments are elevated in V_1 to V_3. **C,** By the fifth hospital day, all precordial T waves are inverted, deeply so, in V_2 to V_4. The diagnosis of critical proximal LAD stenosis was made by Lyn Gilliam, RN, MN, CCRN, Columbia, S.C. Arteriography revealed 90% occlusion of the proximal LAD coronary artery.

Note that during pain (C), there is ST segment elevation as the coronary vessel critically narrows or occludes.

Time Frame for the Development of the Typical ECG

- Present on admission or shortly thereafter in 60% of 180 patients
- Developed within 24 hours in the majority of the remainder of patients
- Developed within 2 to 5 days in a few patients

Emergency Angiography

Because patients with Wellens syndrome without intervention may be imminently destined for massive anterior wall MI, emergency angiography to identify candidates for early revascularization is justified.

Left Main and Three-Vessel Disease
ECG Recognition

I	II	III
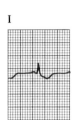	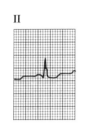	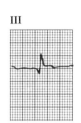

R	L	F
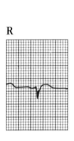	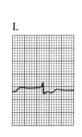	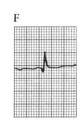

V$_1$	V$_2$	V$_3$
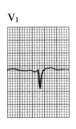	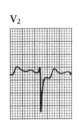	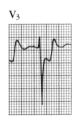

V$_4$	V$_5$	V$_6$
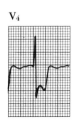	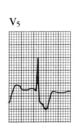	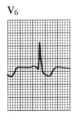

Left main and three-vessel coronary artery disease can be diagnosed in patients with the following characteristics:
- Unstable angina
- ST elevation in aV_R and V_1
- ST depression in 8 or more leads

Management

Emergency arteriography is indicated. The patient may be a candidate for emergency percutaneous transvenous coronary angioplasty (PTCA) or for coronary artery bypass graft (CABG).

⩗ Unstable Angina

Unstable angina is cardiac pain caused by severe transient myocardial ischemia secondary to severe coronary narrowing or occlusion.

Type of Pain

- Recent onset
- Sudden worsening of preexisting angina
- Occurs after a pain-free period
- Stuttering recurrence over days and weeks

Identifying Characteristics

- Not "momentary" in duration.
- Occurs at rest or is brought on by minimal exertion, commonly walking or use of the arms.
- Patient may describe "walking through" or "walking off" the pain.
- During pain, blood pressure and heart rate are usually elevated, S3 gallop is heard, and patient resists lying down.
- Relieved by sublingual nitroglycerin within a few minutes (less than five).

Anginal Pain

Anginal pain may radiate to the following areas:
- Any region above the waist
- Epigastric location (may confuse the diagnosis)
- Most characteristic location: Medial aspect of arms and the mandible
- Retrosternal area (highly specific)
  Note: Localization of the pain to small areas is unusual.

Patients' Common Descriptions of Anginal Pain

- Tightness, heaviness, squeezing, choking, aching, burning, a weight, or numbness
- "Lasts about 2 minutes" (patients tend to overestimate)
- Builds up gradually, plateaus, and subsides gradually

Pain That Is Not Anginal

- After, rather than during, exertion
- Caused by talking
- Caused by "lying on the left side"
- After, rather than during, coitus
- Precipitated exclusively by emotion
- Associated with palpitations, precordial tenderness, lightheadedness, or dysphagia
- "Sharp" (anginal pain is not sticking or needle-like)

Pathogenesis

- Plaque fissure
- Exposure of endothelial collagen and its prothrombotic substrates to flowing blood
- Platelet aggregation
- Release of a vasospastic substance
- Coagulation and thrombus formation

Bundle Branch Block and Hemiblock

25

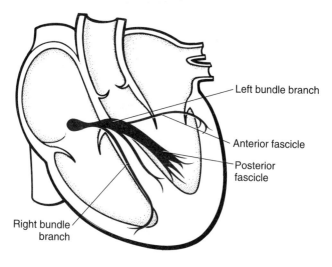

- Left bundle branch
- Anterior fascicle
- Posterior fascicle
- Right bundle branch

The trifascicular specialized conduction system consists of right bundle branch (RBB) and left bundle branch (LBB) with its two main fascicles (anterior and posterior). A block at the level of the right or left bundle causes the ventricles to be activated in sequence instead of simultaneously. This produces a broad QRS complex that has a typical morphology in V_1 and V_6. A block of one of the divisions of the LBB is called *hemiblock*.

Blood Supply

Left anterior descending (LAD) coronary artery supplies: Anterior wall of the heart, anterior two-thirds of the septum, proximal RBB, anterior division of the LBB, part of the posterior division of the LBB.

Right coronary artery supplies (in 90% of individuals): Partly the posterior division of the LBB, posterior one-third of the septum, His bundle (AV nodal branch).

Pediatrics

When found in conjunction with congenital cardiac abnormalities, BBB is usually not accompanied by heart disease and has an excellent prognosis.

T Wave Changes in BBB

Secondary T wave changes: The T wave is opposite in polarity to the terminal component of the QRS complex. If the direction of the T wave is the same as that of the terminal component of the QRS complex, myocardial disease is suspected.

RBBB

Mechanism without MI

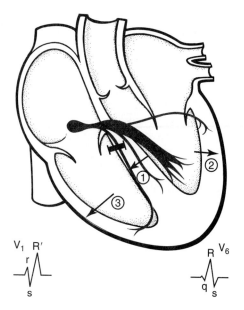

In RBBB, activation of both ventricles in sequence causes a broad complex with a late R wave in V_1 and an S wave in V_6.

1. Normal septal activation: initial r wave in V_1 and a little q wave in lead V_6
2. Normal left ventricular activation: S wave in V_1 and an R wave in V_6
3. Late abnormal right ventricular activation: a late R wave in V_1 and an S wave in V_6

Mechanism with MI

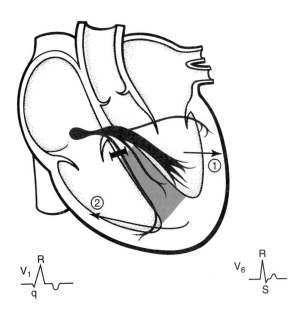

RBBB with MI (QR in V₁)

1. Absent septal activation (necrotic tissue). Left ventricular activation: Q wave in V_1.
2. Late and abnormal right ventricular activation: R wave in V_1

Pattern Variations

V_1

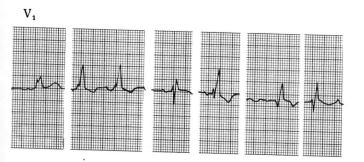

Different patterns of RBBB in V_1. The late R wave is common to all.

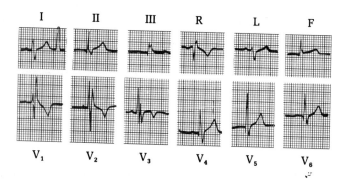

RBBB without MI

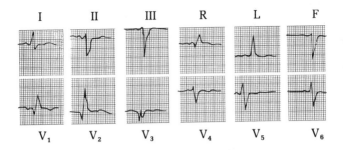

RBBB with anteroseptal MI; anterior hemiblock is also present.

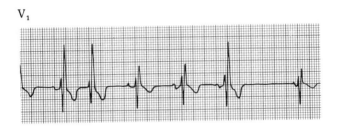

Incomplete RBBB

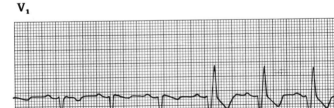

Rate-related RBBB (rate increases from 80–82 beats/min)

Bedside Diagnosis

Complete RBBB: Persistent splitting of S_2

▶ Clinical Implications

- Signifies an occlusion in the proximal LAD coronary artery and extensive myocardial damage
- High chance of developing complete AV block
- High mortality (from pump failure)
- Mortality unaffected by preexisting BBB

Treatment

1. Thrombolytic therapy; if unsuccessful, proceed with the following steps.
2. Emergency PTCA. Insert a Swan-Ganz catheter to gain information about pump function.
3. After reperfusion, if the BBB or fascicular block persists, try temporary prophylactic pacing.

LBBB

Mechanism without MI

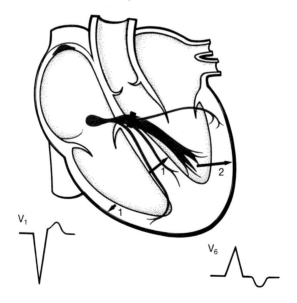

Activation of both ventricles in sequence causes a very broad QRS that is negative in V_1 and totally positive in V_6.

Mechanism with MI

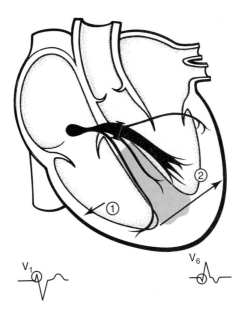

1. Absent septal activation (necrotic tissue). Unopposed right ventricular activation: tall thin R wave in V_1 and a Q wave in V_5 and V_6
2. Left ventricular activation: deep S wave in V_1 and an R wave in V_6

Pattern Variations

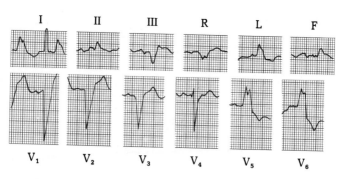

LBBB without MI

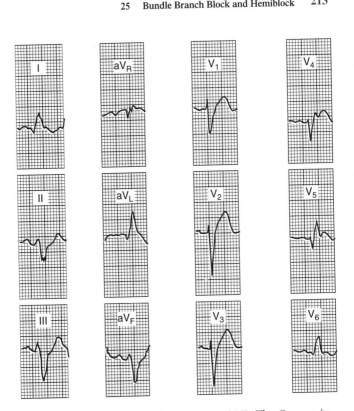

Left bundle branch block and anteroseptal MI. The Q wave in lead V_5 and V_6 and the R wave in lead V_1 are evident.

(From Lyon LJ: Basic electrocardiography handbook, New York, 1977, Van Nostrand Reinhold.)

LBBB with anteroseptal MI

V_1

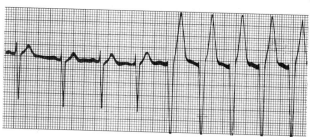

Rate-related LBBB

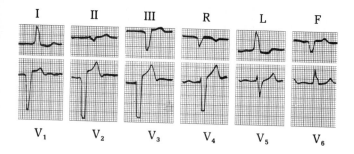

| I | II | III | R | L | F |

| V_1 | V_2 | V_3 | V_4 | V_5 | V_6 |

LBBB with left axis deviation occurs about 30% of the time and is thought to indicate more extensive damage to the anterior fascicle of the left bundle.

V_1

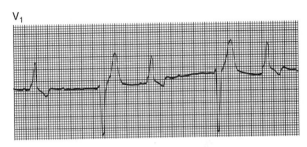

Alternating LBBB and RBBB. In the first four beats, there is RBBB. The left bundle is able to conduct as long as the rate is slow enough. When the rate speeds up, the left bundle blocks, unmasking the slow conduction through the right bundle branch (note the long PR interval with the LBBB beats). The next P wave blocks in both bundles, and the sequence begins again: (1) a short PR interval and conduction over the left bundle (RBBB). (2) block in the left bundle and slow conduction over the right bundle (LBBB with a long PR interval), and (3) block in both bundles.
Courtesy Hein J. Wellens, M.D., Maastricht, The Netherlands.

An alternating LBBB and RBBB indicates disease in both bundles.

Bedside Diagnosis

Complete LBBB: Reversed splitting of S_2

Clinical Implications

The physician should be notified if LBBB develops in the setting of acute anteroseptal MI. The prognosis depends on the underlying cause.

Treatment

None, although in the setting of acute anteroseptal MI, a pacemaker may be indicated.

ECG Recognition of Underlying Cardiac Disease

Axis: 0 degrees or left.
P wave: Left atrial enlargement.
Before onset of LBBB: Abnormal ECG.

Comparison of Lead V_1 in RBBB and LBBB

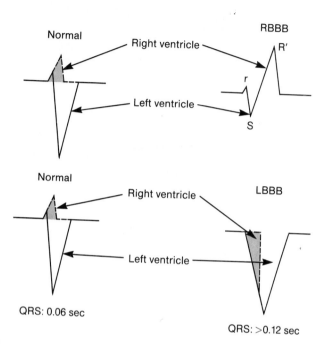

Normal

Right ventricle

Left ventricle

RBBB

R'

r

S

Normal

Right ventricle

Left ventricle

LBBB

QRS: 0.06 sec

QRS: >0.12 sec

Anterior Hemiblock

Anterior hemiblock is a block of the anterior superior division of the LBB.

Mechanism

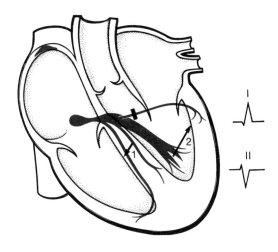

1. Septal and inferior initial forces: q wave in I and aV$_L$
2. Left ventricular activation from the posterior fascicle: left axis deviation

ECG Characteristics

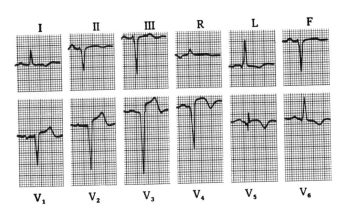

Distinguishing features:
- Left axis deviation of more than −45 degrees
- Terminal R wave in aV_R and aV_L
- R wave in aV_r later than the R wave in aV_L
- q wave in I and aV_L
- r wave in II, III, and aV_F
- Increased QRS voltage in the limb leads

Causes

- Found in otherwise normal hearts
- Lenegre's disease
- Lev's disease
- Aortic valve calcification
- Cardiomyopathy
- Ischemic heart disease
- Acute MI
- Cardiac catheterization
- Selective coronary arteriography
- Hyperkalemia
- Surgical correction of tetralogy of Fallot

▶ Clinical Implications

The physician should be notified of the development of anterior hemiblock. The prognosis depends on the underlying cause.

Pattern Variations

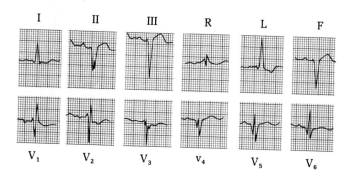

RBBB and anterior hemiblock

II

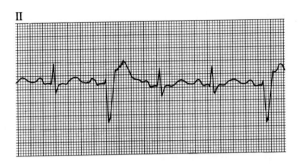

Intermittent anterior hemiblock with first-degree AV block and RBBB

Treatment

Usually none. In the setting of acute anteroseptal MI, a pacemaker may be indicated.

Posterior Hemiblock

Posterior hemiblock is a block of the posterior division of the LBB.

Mechanism

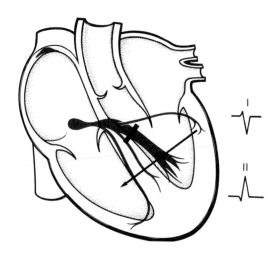

1. Upward and leftward initial forces: r wave in I and II and a q wave in II, III, and aV_F
2. Rightward terminal forces: marked right axis deviation

ECG Characteristics

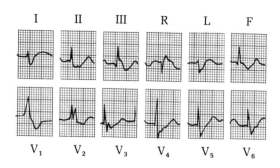

Distinguishing features:
- Right axis deviation of greater than +120 degrees
- q wave in II, III, and aV_F

- r wave in I and aV$_L$
- Increased QRS voltage in the limb leads

Causes

- Lenegre's disease
- Lev's disease
- Aortic valve calcification
- Cardiomyopathy
- Ischemic heart disease
- Acute MI
- Cardiac catheterization
- Selective coronary arteriography
- Hyperkalemia

Clinical Implications

The physician should be notified if posterior hemiblock develops. In the setting of acute anteroseptal MI, posterior hemiblock is associated with RBBB and carries a poor prognosis; complete subnodal AV block develops in 90% of cases.

Trifascicular Block

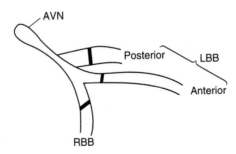

Trifascicular block. *AVN,* Atrioventricular node.

Trifascicular block is located simultaneously (complete or incomplete) in the three main fascicles of the intraventricular conduction system, the RBB, and the anterior and posterior divisions of the LBB.

ECG Recognition

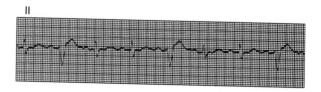

Anterior hemiblock every third beat; prolonged PR interval and QRS duration

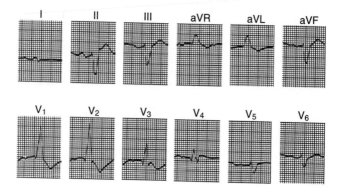

Same patient, later. Anterior wall MI, anterior hemiblock (left axis), RBBB, long PR interval. Three fascicles are involved.

Summary of ECG Recognition of BBB and Hemiblock

RBBB	LBBB	LAH	LPH

WITHOUT MI

WITH MI

LAH, Left anterior hemiblock; *LBBB,* left bundle branch block; *LPH,* left posterior hemiblock; *MI,* myocardial infarction; *RBBB,* right bundle branch block.

Acute Myocardial Infarction

26

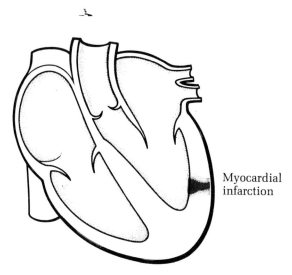

Myocardial infarction

Myocardial infarction (MI) progresses acutely through ischemia and injury, which are reversible, to necrosis, which is not. The pathology is reflected by inverted, symmetrical T waves (ischemia), elevated ST segments (acute injury), and pathological Q waves (necrosis) in the ECG leads over the infarct.

Pathophysiology of the Evolving MI

The underlying pathophysiology of acute MI is the atherosclerotic plaque. The *initiating event* in acute MI is the plaque rupture, platelet aggregation, fibrin deposition, spasm, and thrombus formation. Cellular pathology following coronary occlusion produces life-threatening ventricular arrhythmias, especially in the first 15 to 30 minutes.

ECG Signs of MI

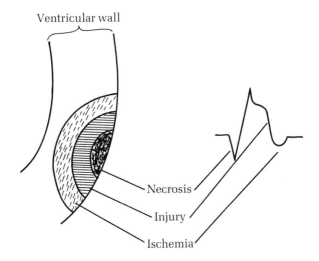

Ventricular wall

Necrosis

Injury

Ischemia

- T wave changes (usually inversion) appear almost immediately (5–30 min).
- ST segment elevation is visible.
- Abnormal Q waves may appear as early as 2 hr from the onset of chest pain. These signify abnormal electrical activity but not necessarily irreversible myocardial damage.

Note:
  - ST segment elevation and Q waves are seen in only about one-half of acute MI cases on presentation.
  - Approximately one-fourth of patients with acute MI do not present with classic chest pain.
  - About one-half of patients presenting with chest pain who ultimately have acute MI have nondiagnostic ECGs on admission.

Diagnostic Leads

Anterior	V_3 and V_4
Anteroseptal	V_1 to V_4
Lateral	I, aV_L, and V_6
Anterolateral	I, aV_L, and V_3 to V_6
Extensive anterior	I, aV_L, and V_1 to V_6
High lateral	I and aV_L
Inferior	II, III, aV_F
Inferoposterior	II, III, aV_F; reciprocal changes precordial leads
Right ventricular	V_{4R} (ST elevation)
Atrial	I, II, III, V_1, V_2, V_5, V_6

Anterior Wall MI

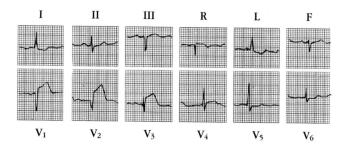

Anteroseptal MI

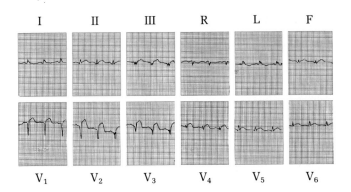

Anterolateral MI

ECG Identification of High-Risk Patients

- BBB
- Hemiblock
- Type II second-degree AV block

Pathology

- Proximal LAD coronary artery occlusion
- May be combined lesion of the LAD and RCA or left circumflex artery
- May extend from the anterior wall into the septum (anteroseptal infarction) and to the left base, free wall, or apex

Inferior MI

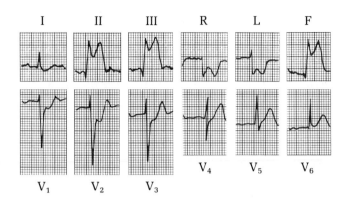

Inferoposterior MI

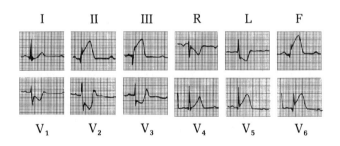

Inferoposterolateral MI

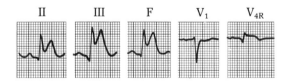

Inferior and right ventricular MI

ECG Identification of High-Risk Patients

- ST elevation in lead V_{4R}
- Complete AV block
- Anterior precordial ST depression
- Lateral ST elevation

Pathology

Right coronary artery occlusion: Inferior posterior MI.
Circumflex occlusion: Inferior lateral MI.

Value of Lead V_{4R} in Locating the Occluded Artery

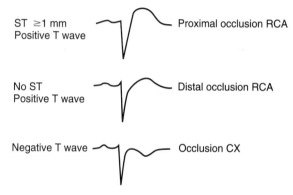

ST ≥1 mm
Positive T wave — Proximal occlusion RCA

No ST
Positive T wave — Distal occlusion RCA

Negative T wave — Occlusion CX

Three possible patterns in lead V_{4R} in patients during the early hours of acute inferior MI. These patterns identify the location of the occlusion. *RCA,* Right coronary artery; *CX,* circumflex coronary artery.

From Wellens HJJ, Conover M: *The ECG in emergency decision making,* Philadelphia, 1991, WB Saunders.

Value of Leads II and III in Locating the Occluded Artery

RCA occlusion: ST segment elevation in III greater than in II.
Circumflex occlusion: ST segment elevation in II greater than in III.

Right Ventricular MI

ECG Diagnosis

ST segment elevation of greater than or equal to 1 mm in V_{4R}

▶ Clinical Implications

- Serious hemodynamic consequences.
- Present in 19 to 51% of patients with acute inferior MI.
- A strong, independent prognostic parameter for life-threatening postinfarction tachyarrhythmias, AV block (45%), and acute and long-term outcome after inferior MI.
- Early diagnosis of RV infarction avoids mismanagement.
- Diuretics, nitroglycerin, and morphine decrease preload.
- In patients who have hemodynamic compromise, knowledgeable medical treatment and informed hemodynamic monitoring help to avoid acute tamponade from RV volume overload squeezing the LV.
- Early diagnosis allows anticipation of conduction problems and arrhythmias, which are aggressively treated.

Inferolateral MI

ECG Recognition

ST segment elevation, Q waves, and inverted T waves in the inferior leads (II, III, aV_F) and in the leads reflecting the lateral wall, such as I and aV_L (high lateral wall!), and V_5 and V_6.

ECG Identification of High-Risk Patients

1. ST elevation in lead $V4_R$ (proximal RCA occlusion and right ventricular infarction)
2. Complete AV block
3. Anterior precordial ST depression (posteroseptal involvement)

Atrial Infarction

ECG Recognition

- PR segment
  - Elevation greater than 0.5 mm in V_5 and V_6 with PR segment depression in V_1 and V_2, or
  - Elevation greater than 0.5 mm in lead I with PR segment depression in II and III, or
  - Depression greater than 1.5 mm in precordial leads and greater than 1.2 mm in leads I, II, and III combined with atrial arrhythmias.
- P wave shapes: W-shaped, M-shaped, notched, or irregular

Clinical Implications

- Occurs in 7–17% of MI (necropsy findings)
- Supraventricular arrhythmias often complicate atrial infarctions

Other Causes of PR Segment Depression

- Pericarditis
- Sympathetic stimulation
- Atrial overloading due to left ventricular failure

Molecular Serum Markers in the Diagnosis of Acute MI

- Creatine kinase (CK) isoenzymes (MM, BB, and MB)
- MM-CK tissue isoform
- MB-CK tissue isoform
- Myoglobin (more rapidly released than CK and CK-MB)
- Cardiac-specific troponins (cTnI and cTnT) (more cardiac-specific than CK-MB)
- Lactic dehydrogenase (LDH)

Emergency Response

- Thrombolytic therapy[1]
- Primary PTCA[1]

Signs of Successful Reperfusions

- Early transient elevation of ST segment; may not be noted
- Rapid reduction in ST segment elevation; frequently preceded by transient elevation; followed by rapid development of pathologic Q wave and loss of R wave amplitude
- Relief of chest pain
- Early T wave inversion

---

[1]Ryan TJ, Anderson JL, Antman EM, Braniff BA, Brooks NH, Califf RM, Hillis LD, Hiratzka LF, Rapaport E, Riegel BJ, Russell RO, Smith EE III, Weaver D: ACC/AHA guidelines for the management of patients with acute myocardial infarction: A report of the American College of Cardiology/American Heart Association Task Force on Practice Guidelines (Committee on Management of Acute Myocardial Infarction), *J Am Coll Cardiol* 28:1328, 1996.

- Early peak of serum CK levels
- Reperfusion arrhythmias

Signs of Partial Reperfusion

- Partial resolution of ST segment
- Increasing mortality risk over long term
- May benefit from vigorous adjunctive pharmacotherapy

Signs of No Reperfusion

- Lack of resolution of ST segment
- Poor prognosis
- May benefit from emergency PTCA or intracoronary thrombolysis

T Wave Inversions Not Caused by MI

- Ischemia of unstable angina
- Following periods of abnormal depolarization (VT, WPW syndrome, and LBBB)
- Normal variant
- Cerebrovascular accident
- Acute pulmonary embolism
- Artifact

ST-T Changes Not Caused by MI

- Prinzmetal's angina (reversible severe coronary artery spasm; characterized by chest pain and ST elevation that quickly reverts to normal)
- Left main and three-vessel disease (unstable angina; diffuse ST depression with ST elevation in aV_R and V_1; usually during pain)
- Critical proximal LAD stenosis (unstable angina; progressive deep symmetrical T wave inversion in V_2 and V_3; without pain)
- Acute pulmonary embolism
- Ventricular aneurysm
- Pericarditis
- Artifact

Nonspecific ST-T Changes

- Minor ST segment deviations
- Flattening of the T wave
- Slight T wave inversions

Q Waves from Causes Other Than MI

- Normal variant
- Acute pulmonary embolism
- Infiltrative myocardial disease
- Intraventricular conduction problems
- Ventricular hypertrophy

Guidelines for the Management of Acute MI[1]

Initial Evaluation

1. Clinical examination and a 12-lead ECG within 10 minutes
2. Door-to-needle time less than 30 minutes

Upon Arrival in Emergency Department

1. Oxygen by nasal prongs
2. Sublingual nitroglycerin (unless systolic arterial pressure is <90 mm Hg or heart rate is <50 or >100 bpm)
3. Adequate analgesia (morphine sulfate or meperidine)
4. Aspirin (160–325 mg orally and continued indefinitely)
5. Intravenous access
6. Continuous ECG monitoring

12-Lead ECG

1. Obtained and interpreted within 10 minutes of arrival in the Emergency Department.
2. ST segment elevation greater than or equal to 1 mV in 2 or more contiguous leads or left bundle branch block (LBBB) and symptoms of acute MI: Immediate fibrinolysis or primary PTCA.
3. Symptoms of acute MI and LBBB are managed like ST segment elevation.
4. Patients without ST segment elevation do not receive thrombolytic therapy.
5. Hospitalization period following fibrinolysis the same as for ST elevation or new LBBB without fibrinolysis.

---

[1]See footnote on page 231.

Acute Pulmonary Embolism

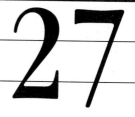

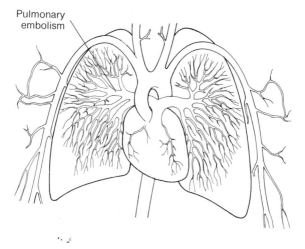

Pulmonary embolism

Massive acute pulmonary embolism (APE) is a devastating clinical entity often undiscovered until autopsy. Acute right ventricular failure may progress to death within minutes to hours after the embolic event. Prompt diagnosis and treatment are imperative, but they may be delayed by clinical instability. Diagnosis is based on clinical suspicion, ventilation-perfusion scanning, ECG signs, and echocardiography.

Common ECG Findings in the Acute Phase

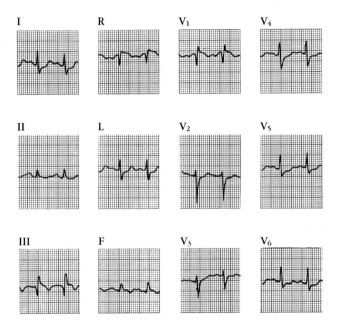

The common ECG findings in APE are the result of right ventricular failure and acute dilation of the right atria and right ventricle.

- Complete or incomplete RBBB
- P-pulmonale
- S wave in leads I and aVL (>1.5 mm or an R:S ratio of <1)
- Transitional zone shifts left
- Q waves in III and aVF
- Frontal plane QRS axis shifts to the right by 20 degrees or more
- T wave inversion in leads III and aV_F or in V_1 to V_4 (a late sign)
- Arrhythmias—sinus tachycardia, atrial fibrillation, atrial flutter, PACs (right atrial), and PVCs (right ventricular)
- ST elevation in aV_R, V_1, III

Pathophysiology

In APE, a central or peripheral pulmonary artery is suddenly obstructed. Acute right ventricular failure may progress to death within minutes to hours after the embolic event. Significant obstruction results in the following pathophysiology:

- Acute pulmonary hypertension
- Right-side dilatation
- Clockwise cardiac rotation
- Right ventricular failure
- Pulmonary infarction
- Marked ventilation-perfusion disturbance
- Acute lowering of the cardiac output

Signs and Symptoms

- Tachypnea
- Dyspnea
- Chest pain
- Sinus tachycardia
- Syncope or near-syncope
- Hepatomegaly
- Palpable right ventricular impulse
- Increase in jugular venous a wave
- Increase in jugular venous distention
- Palpable pulmonary artery pulsation

Physical Findings

Physical findings are related to acute right ventricular volume overload, right ventricular failure, and the increase in pulmonary artery pressure:

- Tricuspid regurgitation
- Audible right ventricular S_4
- S_3 heart sound
- Narrow splitting of S_2 with an exaggerated P_2
- Pulmonary ejection murmur

Common Risk Factors

- Old age
- Prior thromboembolism

- Immobility
- Cancer
- Chronic disease
- Congestive heart failure
- Pelvic and lower extremity surgery
- Varicosities
- Obesity
- Use of oral contraceptives
- Hypertension
- Diabetes mellitus
- Atrial fibrillation
- Hyperlipidemia

Treatment

1. Immediately begin oxygen, analgesics, and heparin therapy. As needed, provide intubation and mechanical ventilation.
2. Massive APE with hypotension or shock is treated with thrombolytic drugs in the absence of contraindications.
3. Surgical embolectomy for APE is controversial, but it appears to have a role for unstable APE when there are absolute contraindications to thrombolysis or when thrombolytic therapy fails.
4. Hypotension may be relieved by preload reduction (norepinephrine [Levophed]) or even by gentle diuresis.
5. Use caution with intravenous fluids (the condition of a hypotensive patient with right ventricular overload from APE usually is made worse by a fluid challenge).
6. Various intrapulmonary arterial catheter techniques, with or without low-dose thrombolytic therapy, have been used successfully to reduce the embolic burden.

   Note: Closed-chest CPR is ineffective when the pulmonary circulation is obstructed by thrombus. Emergency thoracotomy or femorofemoral cardiopulmonary bypass is used in patients with full cardiac arrest from APE.

Prevention

Prevention of deep venous thrombosis, common after all surgical procedures, is fundamental in the prevention of APE.

- Low-dose heparin
- Low-molecular-weight heparin
- Graduated compression elastic stockings
- Intermittent pneumatic compression
- Oral anticoagulants

Hypertrophy

28

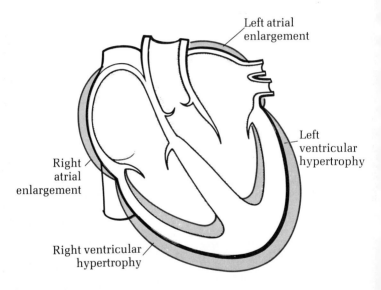

Ventricular hypertrophy results from increased metabolic demands or increased work load because of pressure overload (as in aortic stenosis or systemic hypertension), volume overload (increased end diastolic wall stress), and neurohumoral factors.

Left Ventricular Hypertrophy (LVH)
ECG Recognition (limited sensitivity)

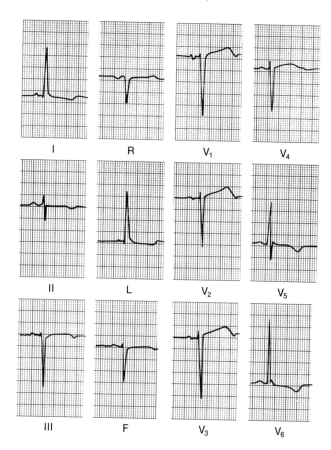

Distinguishing features:
- Tallest precordial R waves in the left chest leads
- Deepest precordial S waves in the right chest leads
- Increased QRS amplitude
- Late intrinsicoid deflection in V_6 (measured from the onset of the QRS to the peak of the R wave)

- Widened QRS/T angle in V_5 and V_6 (left ventricular strain); associated with long-standing LVH and intensifies when dilatation and failure develop
- Tendency toward left axis deviation
- Associated left atrial enlargement

Estes Scoring System for LVH

Points

0.04 sec

− 1.0 mm

0.04 sec × − 1.0 mm = − 0.04 (abnormal)

0.05 sec or more

1. Voltage criteria **3**
   Any of the following:
   a. R or S wave in limb leads = 20 mm
   b. S wave in V_1 or V_2 = 30 mm
   c. R wave in V_5 or V_6 = 30 mm
2. ST-T abnormalities
   Without digitalis **3**
   With digitalis **1**
3. Left atrial abnormality **3**
   Negative area under P wave in lead $V_1 \geq 1$ mm² (1 box)
4. Left axis deviation **2**
5. QRS duration **1**
   − .09 sec
6. Intrinsicoid deflection **1**
   V_5 or $V_6 \geq .05$ sec

*5 Points, diagnostic; 4 points, probable.

Pathophysiology

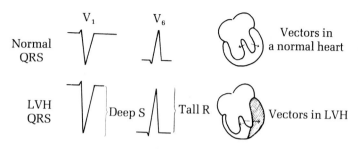

- The normal QRS compared with that in LVH

When the left ventricular wall hypertrophies, the disproportion in size between the left and right ventricles is increased, resulting in greater QRS amplitude. However, a normal sequence of depolarization is retained.

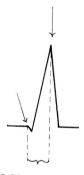

0.05 sec or more

- The intrinsicoid deflection in V_6

The peak of the R wave in V_6 reflects the time it takes for peak voltage to develop under that electrode. Because there is more muscle mass, this deflection is delayed.

▶ Clinical Implications

LVH is causally related to high blood pressure. Its presence in hypertensive patients points to hypertensive target organ damage. When the ECG shows evidence of LVH, there is an associated increased risk for a number of cardiovascular diseases including myocardial infarction, stroke, and congestive heart failure.

Causes

- Hypertension
- Aortic stenosis
- Aortic insufficiency
- Coarctation of the aorta
- Hypertrophic cardiomyopathy
- Athletics
- Myocardial infarction

Treatment

That of the primary disease.

Right Ventricular Hypertrophy (RVH)

ECG Recognition

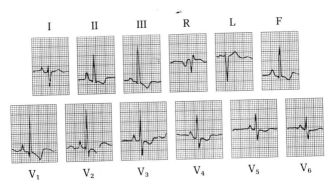

Distinguishing features:
- Right axis deviation of greater than +110 degrees in adults
- Right axis deviation of greater than 120 degrees in the young
- S_1, S_2, S_3 pattern in children
- Late intrinsicoid deflection in V_1 and V_2
- Incomplete RBBB pattern in V_1
- ST segment depression with upward convexity and inverted T waves in V_1 and V_2 and in the limb leads; tall R waves

- Reversal of precordial lead R wave progression (tall R waves in the right precordial leads and deep S waves in the left precordial leads)
- Strain patterns in V_1, V_2, II, III, and aV_F
- Tall, peaked P waves in leads II, III, and aV_F, and sometimes in V_1 (right atrial involvement)
- Slight increase in QRS duration
- Secondary ST-T abnormalities in the precordial and inferior leads (the T wave is opposite in polarity to the QRS)

Pathophysiology

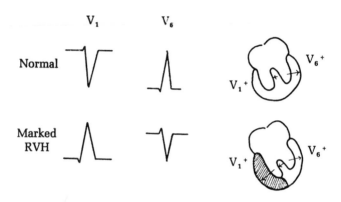

- The normal QRS is compared with that in RVH

   Normally the electrical forces of the thicker left ventricle dominate those of the right ventricle so that an rS appears in V_1 and a qR in V_5 and V_6. In marked right ventricular hypertrophy, the right ventricle dominates, producing characteristic ECG findings.

▶ Clinical Implications

- Congenital pulmonary stenosis
- Tetralogy of Fallot
- Primary pulmonary hypertension

Chronic Obstructive Lung Disease

ECG Recognition

- P waves: Peaked leads II, III, and aV_F (amplitude increases with the severity of the disease); right axis
- QRS complex:
  - Low R wave amplitude (<0.5 mV in V_6 as the disease progresses)
  - Wide slurred S waves in leads I, II, III, and V_4 to V_6
  - In severe disease, R/S ratio is less than or equal to 1 in V_6
- Associated emphysema: Low ECG voltage; posterior and superior QRS axis; P wave axis right of +60 degrees in the frontal plane
- Associated RVH: Right axis deviation; dominant S wave in precordial leads; RBBB pattern in right precordial leads; slurred S wave in left precordial leads; prominent R wave in lead aV_R

Pathophysiology

- Overaerated lungs provide an insulating effect
- Spatial orientation of the heart changes

Biventricular Hypertrophy
ECG Recognition

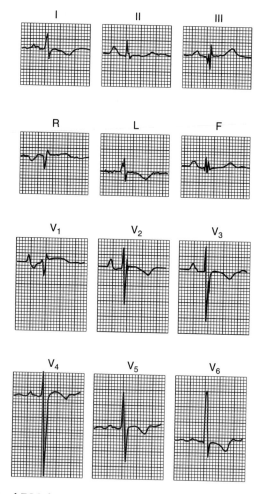

A 12-lead ECG from a patient with hypertension. The notched, upright P wave in leads I, II, and V_4 to V_6 and the deep, broad terminal trough in lead V_1 are evident.

Courtesy Ara G. Tilkian, M.D., Van Nuys, California.

A patient with bilateral disease and probable biventricular hypertrophy. Note P waves (notched in I, II, and V_4 to V_6) and deep broad terminal trough in lead V_1.

- Right axis deviation is present.
- Signs of LVH are visible in the precordial leads.
- The transitional zone shifts to the left (a less-reliable sign).
- When there is hypertrophy of both ventricles, the ECG may be normal.

Clinical Implications

- Eisenmenger's syndrome (ventricular septal defect or patent ductus arteriosus and pulmonary hypertension)

Left Atrial Enlargement; P-Mitrale

- ECG pattern often present in hypertension and may transiently occur in pulmonary edema

ECG Recognition

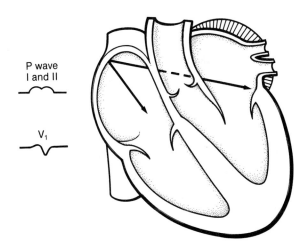

Distinguishing features (P-mitrale):
- Prolonged P wave duration
- Notched upright P wave in I, II, and V_4 to V_6
- Deep, broad terminal trough in V_1

Causes

- Those of LVH

⌁ Right Atrial Abnormality: P-Pulmonale
ECG Recognition

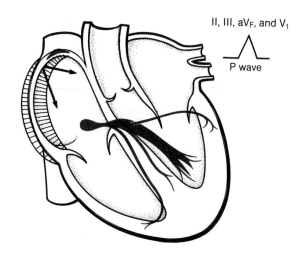

Distinguishing features (P pulmonale)
- Tall peaked P waves in leads II, III, aV$_F$, and sometimes V$_1$
- P axis to the right of +70 degrees.

Pathophysiology

- Increased sympathetic stimulation (causing increased P amplitude)
- Low position of the diaphragm (causing the P axis to be rightward)
- Diffuse lung disease.

▶ Clinical Implications

The P-pulmonale pattern is most helpful in the evaluation of the severity of chronic obstructive lung disease (rightward P axis shift).

Right Atrial Hypertrophy

ECG Recognition

- Tall, wide P waves in the limb leads and right precordial leads
- Often associated with RVH

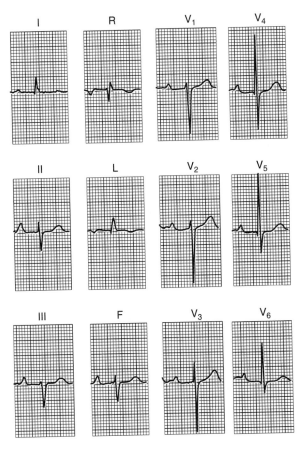

Courtesy Ara G. Tilkian, M.D., Van Nuys, California.

Right atrial hypertrophy caused by tricuspid valve disease (or pulmonary hypertension). Note the tall, wide P waves in the inferior leads and right precordial leads.

Causes

- Congenital heart disease
- Tricuspid valve disease
- Pulmonary hypertension

Expert Bedside Monitoring

Diagnostic monitoring leads

Digitalis Intoxication	PSVT		Unstable Angina	VT	High-risk MI
					Inferior, V_{4R}; Anterior V_1, I, and II
II and/or V_1	I, II, III, V_1, and V_6		V_2 or V_3 $\bar{s}$ pain	V_1, V_2, and V_6	Inferior
II: P in atrial tachycardia	CMT	AVNRT		V_1 positive complex	V_{4R}
			Critical proximal LAD stenosis (Wellens syndrome)	V_1	Proximal RCA occlusion RV MI
If: No conduction or atrial fibrillation			12-lead $\bar{c}$ pain	V_1 need V_6	
			ST ↑ V_1 and a V_R St ↓ Eight other leads	R:S<1 V_1 negative complex V_1 and V_2	Anterior V_1 I II or
			Left main or three-vessel coronary artery disease	V_6	

Copyright 1992 by Mary H. Conover.
AVNRT, Atrioventricular nodal reentry tachycardia; *CMT,* circus movement tachycardia; *c̄,* with; *LAD,* left anterior descending (coronary artery); *MI,* myocardial infarction; *PSVT,* premature supraventricular tachycardia; *RCA,* right coronary artery; *RV,* right ventricular; *s̄,* without; *VT,* ventricular tachycardia.

The ideal monitoring protocol would be to monitor in all 12 leads continuously. However, if this is not possible, the mandatory diagnostic leads are individualized to the patient's clinical condition.

Digitalis Toxicity

Lead II: P waves resemble sinus P waves during atrial tachycardia.
Lead V_1 or MCL_1: Determines ventricular rhythm when there is no conduction or no P waves; junctional rhythm has normal rS pattern; fascicular VT has RBBB pattern.

251

PSVT

Leads I, II, III, V_1, and V_6: Multiple leads during the tachycardia to locate the P' waves, which are not always visible in every lead. P's will be part of the QRS in AV nodal reentry tachycardia (not seen or pseudo-S wave in II and III; pseudo-R wave in V_1). P's follow the QRS in circus movement tachycardia using an accessory pathway.

Unstable Angina

All patients with chest pain are monitored in V_2 or V_3.
During chest pain, all 12 leads are recorded.
- Progressive, deep, symmetrical, T wave inversion indicates critical proximal LAD stenosis.
- ST depression in 8 leads and ST elevation in aV_R and V_1 indicates left main or three-vessel disease.

Broad QRS Tachycardia

V_1, V_2, and V_6
- When V_1 is positive, a monophasic or biphasic pattern indicates VT, as do two peaks with the initial peak highest. A triphasic pattern (rSR') indicates SVT.
- When V_1 is negative, V_1 and V_2 are used: VT is indicated when there is a broad r (>.03 sec), a slurred S downstroke, a delayed S nadir (>0.06 sec), or a q wave in V_6. SVT is indicated if the r wave in V_1 and V_2 is narrow and the S downstroke is swift and clean.

High-Risk Myocardial Infarction

Inferior MI high-risk assessment: V_{4R}: An elevated ST segment (>1 mm) indicates proximal RCA occlusion, high possibility of AV block, RV MI, and high risk.
Anterior MI high-risk assessment: I, II, and V_1: Axis deviation (leads I and II) and the development of BBB (V_1) indicate high risk and aggressive therapy.

Index

Bold page numbers indicate major discussions.